The Quiet Heart

DR PETER GRUENEWALD is a General Medical Practitioner providing holistic health care at the Helios Medical Centre in Bristol and at the Hale Clinic in London. He has worked in the fields of psychiatric rehabilitation, emotional and behavioural difficulties and stress management since 1986, and is founder of the HeartSpheres approach for the management of emotions and interpersonal development. He is involved in the training of health professionals, teachers and care staff in the United Kingdom, Switzerland and the Philippines.

TERESA HALE founded the Hale Clinic, London in 1987 and has been the Managing Director ever since. She is regarded as one of the World's leading "health visionaries". She has played a major role in the growth of complementary medicine over the last 25 years. Teresa Hale is the author of two books. She is a Philosophy and Economics graduate with a postgraduate degree in Education.

The Quiet Heart

Putting Stress in Its Place

Peter Gruenewald

Floris Books

First published in 2007 by Floris Books
Second printing 2009

British Library CIP Data available

ISBN 978-086315-609-0

Printed in Poland

Disclaimer

The aim of this book is to give you practical tools to manage and transform stress and extreme emotions. Its content is not a substitute for the advice of a trained therapist or doctor. This book does not pretend to diagnose medical conditions, and it makes no recommendations regarding medical treatments for such conditions.

In case of serious trauma or mental health problems these exercises may only be done with the permission or under the guidance of an experienced health professional.

Caution

Should you suffer from the effects of severe trauma, do not attempt to work on any highly traumatic events without the help of a qualified therapist as you may put yourself at risk of re-traumatization and aggravation of your symptoms.

Author's Note

The following products, techniques and services referred to in the text are registered trade names: HeartSpheres®, HeartMath®, Freeze-Framer®, Quick Coherence®, Freeze-Framing®, Attitude Breathing®, Heart-Lock-in®, Cut-Thru® and Nonviolent Communication®.

Contents

Foreword

It happens to all of us — at some point negative emotions rear their ugly head and we wonder what to do with them. Often they will not go away — it is like having flu or a virus within the body we want to expel. How do we go about it? *The Quiet Heart* gives us tools with which to transform our negative thoughts and emotions so we can create a positive outlook and experience the harmony and love which is our birthright.

With certain conditions, it may be essential to consult a health professional; however in many cases the simple tools found in this book can empower people to transform their every day negative thoughts, emotions and actions.

Just as when we use tools of preventative medicine like exercise and good nutrition to keep us physically in good shape, the tools in this book enable us to create positive thoughts, emotions and actions.

The techniques are very integrated in their approach using breathing, visualization, affirmation and imagination techniques to achieve their purpose.

Great emphasis is put on controlling the breathing, which has a very important effect on all the physiological systems, particularly the autonomic nervous system. The control of the breath is combined with effective, powerful visualization techniques to awaken positive feelings, such as calmness, appreciation and confidence. The power of imagination is used to help us to transform negative emotion into positive action and to understand the impact this could have on the resolution of conflict within our everyday lives.

This approach can also be utilized for co-creating our future. Instead of focusing on the outcome of future events, the HeartSpheres approach concentrates on mentally rehearsing processes and skills. We can learn to perceive intuitively the potential of future development that suits not only us but the whole of human and social development without any preconceived ideas. So often we are encouraged to visualize exactly what we think we 'want' for the future, instead of concentrating on how to perceive the potential of human and organizational development and transform ourselves in order to facilitate this development of a greater good.

An interesting side effect of this approach is that by changing how we feel about the 'future,' we can transform how we feel about our 'present.'

Scientific research shows us how meditation and techniques used in this book can transform the neuronal connections in the brain. Neuronal connections created by repeated bouts of anger can be changed into such neural pathways that support the expression of positive emotions like understanding, love, care and appreciation. We now have the tools to transform our mental physiology.

Physicists and others like William Tiller, Dean Radin and Amit Goswami are demonstrating scientifically that our thoughts may have a much more profound effect on our external reality than was previously understood. Many examples are quoted in *The Quiet Heart* where, through a person transforming their own emotions, a potential conflict was able to be resolved harmoniously. The inner thoughts appeared to influence the external reality. If this is so, the techniques in this book have a much larger outreach. They are not just about our own internal transformation, but can influence our family, friends, work and external environment.

This book is about the awakening of the heart. It is so much more than just a physical organ and this book puts us in touch with the love, wisdom and strength found within our heart. The heart is only 22 centimetres from the brain but the two are often seen as existing in different dimensions. *The Quiet Heart* shows how the heart and higher brain can operate together and guide us to act in a more harmonious way.

There is great humanity within *The Quiet Heart* combined with scientific understanding. It draws on the work of Johann Wolfgang Goethe's scientific method, which combines external enquiry with inner experience. In the future we may see more and more scientists embracing this form of scientific enquiry.

The author, Dr Peter Gruenewald, is both a colleague and personal friend and in his work I have always found him to combine an intellectual rigour with deep care and compassion for his patients. The advice in this book is not just based on mental constructs but is put into practice in the author's everyday life. He has always been very committed to the idea that we can transform our thoughts, emotions and actions and has given his patients the tools whereby they can achieve this goal by awakening their hearts.

Teresa Hale
May 2007

Introduction

It is easy to be at sea in today's fast-living, competitive and achievement-geared world, and to feel defeated in a whole range of situations that life seems to throws at us every day. This can often lead us into resignation or despair, with the sense that we are helpless victims of circumstance rather than active co-creators of what happens in our lives. We become alienated from ourselves and our loved ones, life starts to seem empty and meaningless, and we compensate for this through addictive behaviour of various kinds, ranging from shopping to hard drugs.

Through freedom and creativity, coupled with a healthy sense of caring and responsibility it is possible to regain power over our lives. This book will show, in practical ways, how we can free ourselves gradually from often inhibiting and destructive fear, anger, sadness, guilt or despair. Even in the midst of a challenging professional, social and private life, we can find a deeper sense of purpose without losing touch with reality. This creative approach does not sweep the reality of difficulties and problems under the carpet, but accepts them fully in order to use the energy and wisdom locked up in them to bring about real change. The benefits of the effective, easy-to-learn techniques presented here can be felt within days, and will enhance all spheres of life: personal, social and professional.

This book is based on the HeartSpheres approach. It is a highly practical guide to enhancing your personal and professional life, while empowering you to take charge and become the co-creator of your circumstances. It will help you to recognize and fundamentally change your emotional response to events. The techniques described here can transform some of your deeper and often unconscious negative beliefs and attitudes about yourself and your life circumstances.

The HeartSpheres approach supports vitality and wellbeing, and improves physical health and relationships with those around you. It helps relieve the emotional stress that we all encounter in everyday situations, and can transform extreme or negative emotions into positive personal and social skills such as courage, self-confidence, independence, self-motivation and other interpersonal skills.

The approach introduces exercises based on the scientific understanding of the physiology of the breathing process, the heart and the brain, and how they all relate to the development of human consciousness. The exercises draw on the awareness that our heart and right-brain hemisphere are resources of deep intuitive and practical knowledge for developing the power of transformation, caring, compassion, strength and self-determination. While these may seem very 'lofty' qualities, in fact they are core values. The presence or absence of these values profoundly affects everyday life. The way we perceive ourselves and the world — our overall outlook, you might say — exerts a decisive influence for good or ill on the actual course of our lives.

It is, however, not enough just to develop a more 'positive' outlook, for our emotions are also based on physiological patterns which can trigger them involuntarily. These patterns have developed through past interaction, environment and inheritance (genetic factors). Although these factors are often considered as not capable of being changed, they are nevertheless open to recognition and transformation through personal development. The techniques taught here help to master and transform underlying physiological responses and patterns. Learning these skills will deepen self-knowledge and empower you, without the process of lengthy psychotherapy.

What do the exercises involve?

This book introduces seven main HeartSpheres exercises, together with three supplementary exercises. They involve clinically validated techniques such as focused relaxation, controlled rhythmic breathing, visualization, affirmation, Contemplation and generating positive feelings. The exercises are safe, highly effective and easy to learn and apply.

Personalizing the exercises

The way the HeartSpheres exercises are outlined in this book, is based on long personal, coaching and clinical experience. Although it will be initially important to strictly follow the instructions, the author has always encouraged his clients to individualize the exercises, as they develop the confidence to do so. This individualization will make the exercises increasingly personal, helping clients to fully own them and allowing for artistic freedom in the process. Many of the case studies published in this book are excellent examples of an individualized practice.

Summing up the benefits

The HeartSpheres exercises are taught as an effective method of stress management in personal development workshops, individual coaching sessions and as professional development techniques for health professionals and therapists. The techniques can also be very useful in conflict resolution and mediation, and can be complemented by techniques such as the Nonviolent Communication developed by Marshall B. Rosenberg. (see Part 3, p.153).

Since these exercises help to reduce the impact of extreme emotions on our physical, emotional and mental health, they can play an important role in health promotion, prevention and as additional support for the treatment of many stress-related physical and mental health problems, such as anxiety disorder, depression, insomnia, chronic fatigue syndrome, hypertension and irritable bowel syndrome.

The skills learned through the HeartSpheres exercises improve people's daily lives in a wide variety of ways.

Practising the HeartSpheres approach enables us to:

~ learn how to *prevent the damaging effects* of stress by becoming aware of how and when the negative stress response is initiated, how to stop it progressing and finally how to prevent it affecting body and mind;

~ *accept that stress in everyday life* is unavoidable, and begin to meet our own stress with greater equanimity;

~ learn how to *alleviate physical symptoms* associated with stress, such as high blood pressure, cardiovascular disease, irritable bowel syndrome, migraine, chronic pain, sleep disorders and many others;

~ enhance personal and professional development by helping to *transform negative emotions* into positive human qualities, such as courage, enthusiasm, openness, self- confidence, initiative, assertiveness and listening skills;

~ *enhance performance* and improve memory, concentration, focus, decision-making, intuitive assessment and speed of performance;

~ *improve personal relationships* by developing understanding, compassion and forgiveness for oneself and others;

~ *reduce negative emotional response* to current life situations, created by past events that colour our present perceptions and behaviour. Such experiences — that often lie long ago in childhood, and may have been forgotten — can remain with us and cause stressful feelings of all kinds, or can create inappropriate responses to a present difficulty. The exercises given here help transform past traumatic experiences and their influence on present life;

~ *prevent attracting similar traumatic events* again in the future, by creating different patterns of response to situations.

How to use this book

Part 1 contains the actual exercises with guidance for their use, and suggestions about how to derive the most benefit from them. The exercises are presented in logical sequence: each one builds on the one before and enhances it further. I recommend that you start with the Heart Breathing exercise then add the Inner Dialogue to a shortened version of the Heart Breathing exercise after a few weeks. These two exercises can be done during the same exercise session.

The Heart Breathing exercise and the Inner Dialogue exercise can be practised once daily.

All other exercises can be practised any time you feel the need to support or deepen one or another aspect of these core exercises. These are merely guidelines and can of course be adapted to your individual needs and requirements.

Part 2 explores the rationale underlying this practical approach. Clearly it is helpful to understand how and why HeartSpheres techniques work, and what they involve, when embarking on them. A general understanding of these techniques gives an additional impetus for subsequent motivation and practice.

Part 3 explores related approaches that have inspired me in developing the HeartSpheres exercises (the roots). Some of the approaches outlined in Part 3 can complement the HeartSpheres exercises.

Part 1

The Practice

Before you start

As is the case with all relaxation, breathing or meditation exercises, it is vital to remain focused and present. Over time you will certainly become more skilled in your attempts to maintain and deepen focus and relaxation. Be patient with yourself and try to avoid being too goal-orientated. Although you will feel some immediate relief from stress and the impact that negative emotions had on you, when practising the exercises, long-term effects and deep-seated problems will need time to resolve and transform. The very effort of doing the exercises helps us to face life's daily challenges; therefore the emphasis is not on how successfully we manage them, but that we are doing them at all.

Do not practise the exercises for more than thirty minutes at a time. Initially a shorter period of time might be a good idea. For example five to ten minutes — just see what feels right for you. In the beginning you may experience various bodily sensations, which are often an indication that your perception of your body is changing, or coming into sharper focus. Take things slowly, open your eyes during the exercise to regain control and ease the sensations, if needed. Take a break if required, and do not force any of the exercises unless they feel natural to you. Most of these sensations are short-lived and tend to disappear entirely with practice.

During the breathing exercise sensations of mild dizziness can occur. Some disturbing feelings can arise, such as fear and anxiety, which may have been previously suppressed. These are usually of a mild and transient nature and mean that you need to proceed very slowly, gently adapting to the new psychological and physical experiences. At times memory images or imaginative pictures can surface as a result of the deep relaxation process. Sensations of floating and physical weightlessness, increased circulation (warmth) or pins and needles may be experienced. All these experiences are mild and transient, and will stop when the exercise ends.

Perform your exercises gently and do not put yourself under any pressure. Where appropriate perform your exercises with open eyes in order to stay in control of your experiences. Initially it is good to do the exercises in a sitting position so as not to fall asleep.

Please keep the following in mind:

~ How well you do these exercises is less important than the effort you put into them, which in itself has a beneficial effect.

~ Overcoming inner and outer resistance is part of the developmental process. Don't be too self-critical; be kind and compassionate with yourself. You can always make up for a missed exercise another time.

~ Developing new skills takes time and requires patience. Some areas of personal development need more time than others. You will make continual, gradual progress even if you are not always aware of it. However, you are likely to recognize some progress soon after starting to practise these exercises.

~ Regularity and perseverance, combined with sincerity and genuine enjoyment of the exercises, will guarantee progress.

~ Keeping to a rhythm, a certain time of day, helps maintain practice.

Case Study: Preparing a Difficult Meeting

~

The day after I took part in an introductory workshop on the HeartSpheres techniques I attended a meeting about which I was very concerned. I knew a difficult issue would be discussed about which I felt a huge resentment. I was worried that my resentment would get the better of me and that I would create an angry scene. In addition a manager would be present whom I had confronted about lying once before, fuelling my resentment even further.

Ten minutes before the meeting I sat down quietly, did the first part of the Heart Breathing exercise and reminded myself of my experience with the Listening with the Heart exercise. That took five minutes. I then had another five minutes to 'come back into the world' and make my way into the meeting room.

Once there I was amazed at how calm I was and how much genuine appreciation I experienced for the manager's general attitude and professionalism.

When I spoke it felt as if the resentment had simply vanished. Instead I was clear, articulate and assertive when I stated a request. The words just came without premeditation and it was only when I actually spoke that I realized my request meant that it would be difficult for the manager to 'be economical with the truth' at a later point. My request was accepted.

Since then I have practised the HeartSpheres exercises on a daily basis. As a result I am generally calmer and able to quietly and assertively ask for what I want as well as set boundaries. Until now I have had great difficulties with both of these.

M.F., Accountant, aged 49

1. The HeartSpheres Exercises

If I had to limit my advice on healthier living to just one
tip, it would be simply to learn how to breathe correctly.
Improper breathing is a common cause of ill health.

Andrew Weil

The Heart Breathing exercise

The Heart Breathing exercise combines elements of focused
relaxation, visualization, affirmation, and a balancing breathing technique, which gives us access to fully alert states of
extended consciousness, and increases the effectiveness of
subsequent exercises by allowing us to access our higher self
and subconscious mind. Physiologically, it balances our autonomic nervous system, our endocrine (hormonal) function
and strengthens our immune system.

The Heart Breathing exercise helps to develop meditative
and reflective skills, while significantly reducing stress, and
supporting the development of core values such as calmness
and security, caring and appreciation, and strength and confidence. Each of these qualities is addressed individually.
The symbols and affirmations used support the deepening of
the particular experiences. The Heart Breathing exercise is
a very powerful meditation, which leads into deep-focused
relaxation and enhances intuitive insight, empathy and
effectiveness.

All exercises work best if practised regularly in a rhythm
which fits with your life and circumstances. To practise them
at the same time each day reinforces their effect. The time
soon after waking and/or before falling asleep can be par-

ticularly effective. Don't try to do the exercises for at least one hour after a main meal. For further explanations and instructions on breathing, sensualization and affirmation, see The Techniques of Transformation, p.121.

The Heart Breathing exercise consists of the following parts:

~ Balanced Breathing
~ Affirmation of Core Skills:
   — Calmness and security
   — Strength and confidence
   — Caring and appreciation
~ Contemplation
~ Mental Rehearsing

Start with Balanced Breathing and the Affirmation of Core Skills (see below).

The Contemplation and Mental Rehearsing can be added whenever you feel ready. The whole Heart Breathing exercise should not take more than thirty minutes.

With time, the depth of focus and relaxation will increase and the single steps become so familiar that they can be done in only a few minutes without losing their power. The intensity of feeling and intention you manage to generate is more important for the efficacy of the exercise than the time spent.

Balanced Breathing

Balanced Breathing is a technique of slow, regular, whole chest and abdominal breathing that focuses on the relationship between heart (inhalation) and body periphery (exhalation).

~ Make sure that nobody and nothing can disturb you.

~ Sit or lie down and close your eyes. (If you feel uncomfortable closing your eyes, then perform the exercise initially with eyes open.)

~ Breathe relaxation into your body and mind, and breathe away any tension, thoughts or images.

~ Breathe freely through your nose, if possible — try not to control your breathing.

~ With each inhalation gently expand your abdomen and then the middle and upper part of your ribcage. Whilst inhaling expand the back space of your ribcage too, by breathing consciously into it, beginning with the lower back, then slowly moving up to the middle part of the back and the shoulder region. As you progress, maintain awareness of the front and back of the ribcage simultaneously.

~ Exhale slowly and completely and await the urge to inhale again.

~ The inhalation and exhalation should be equally long and slow. Maintain heart breathing throughout the whole exercise. Breathe gently, as you may become dizzy otherwise. Don't force your breath.

~ After you have established a comfortable level of breathing as described above, you can begin to slowly reduce your breathing rhythm to approximately six cycles per minute (inhalation: 4 seconds / break: 1 second / exhalation: 4–5 seconds / break: 1 second). [4:1:4:1]

Inhalation	Pause	Exhalation	Pause
4 seconds	1 second	4 seconds	1 second

~ It may take a few days or as long as a few weeks for the slowness of breathing (six cycles per minute) to feel natural for you. You can start with ten cycles per minute (breathing three seconds in and three seconds out) and then reduce it slowly day by day, or week by week, to six cycles per minute. You can do this by initially counting to 3, 4 or 5 for every inhalation and exhalation or by using a watch (six to ten seconds for every breathing cycle). Don't force the rhythm. The slow breathing has to be gentle and needs to feel natural. Later you will be able to achieve this rhythm naturally as a result of your practice. You will not have to focus too much on your breathing any more. Breathing with six cycles per minute will help you to reduce stress instantly, will deepen relaxation and focus and balance your autonomic nervous system.

~ Try to observe your thoughts, images or emotions rising in a fairly detached manner. Take an interest in them, then send them away and refocus on your breathing and your meditation. Do not get alarmed if emotions or weariness are released as you start to relax.

Then progress to the next steps. Balanced Breathing is maintained throughout the whole exercise.

Affirmation of Core Skills

The following core skills are developed and deepened through the simultaneous use of slow, regular breathing, visualization and a simple, positive statement that is repeated with every breathing cycle:

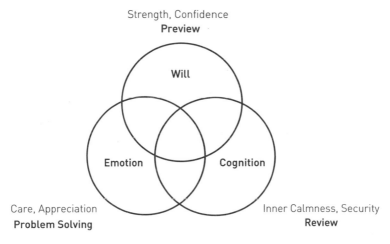

~ *Calmness and security* allow us to detach ourselves from our experience and enhance our capacity for processing experience (*Cognition*).

~ *Strength and confidence* help us to change ourselves and the world around us and enhance our capacity to act, since they enhance the power of the *will*.

~ *Caring and appreciation* for ourselves and others connect us with life, nature, ourselves and our fellow human beings and enhance our capacity to experience the world around us through feeling. They connect and balance the polarities of calmness (*cognition*) and strength (*will*), and self and world.

The core imagination

The influence of the heart doesn't stop with the physical organ in the centre of our chest. Peripheral circulation in arteries, veins and capillaries is intimately related to the activity of the heart. Furthermore the heart is the strongest source of electromagnetic activity within the human body. The electromagnetic field of the heart envelops our entire body and reaches about five feet into the space that surrounds us. This space can also be described as the 'outer'.

The sun is the brightest star in our planetary system, the centre and source of *light, warmth and life* for the earth and the rest of the planetary system. The sunlight is bright, warm and, in moderation, an important source of energy for all life processes.

In this exercise, sunlight symbolizes the qualities of *calmness and security, strength and confidence*, and finally *caring and appreciation*.

Picture yourself surrounded by a sphere filled with golden rays of sunlight. Imagine the brightness, warmth and life-enhancing effect of this sunlight and how it impacts on your body and mind. Picture how sunlight flows from the periphery through your skin, limbs and organs into your heart as you inhale, and how sunlight flows from your heart through your organs and skin into the periphery as you exhale. In your imagination, the heart breathes sunlight as the lungs breathe air.

Creating and sustaining of positive feelings

As you inhale:

- ~ Imagine how feelings of calmness and security are inhaled with the sunlight through the boundaries of your body (skin) into your heart (mid-chest), filling your entire body and heart with sunlight, calmness, peace and security.

~ Hear inwardly the following affirmation as if it is being spoken to you from outside:

«Calm in you»

As you exhale:

~ Imagine sunlight flowing with feelings of calmness and security from your heart through your body and beyond into the periphery (surrounding).

~ Speak inwardly the following affirmation:

«I am calm »

~ The heart is in the centre of both movements: it receives the sunlight and these feelings from our surroundings as we inhale, and sends them out to people in need of support as we exhale.

~ Sustain the feelings of calmness and security whilst hearing (inhalation) and speaking (exhalation) the affirmations inwardly.

~ Maintain simultaneous awareness of the body's centre (heart) and periphery (skin and beyond) throughout both inhalation and exhalation.

~ Repeat the two affirmations at least seven times.

Then move on to the next two core feelings and affirmations and proceed in the same way as above, imagining the core feelings carried by the rays of sunlight. The three core qualities and their affirmations are:

1. Calmness and security
   «Calm in you» (inhalation / hearing)
   «I am calm» (exhalation / speaking)

2. Strength and confidence
   «Strength in you» (inhalation / hearing)
   «I am strong» (exhalation / speaking)

3. Caring and appreciation
   «Care in you» (inhalation / hearing)
   «I am caring» (exhalation / speaking)

Work on each of these feelings for at least seven breathing cycles, but longer is better.

You can add your own affirmations to your meditation if you wish to work on other core values or skills such as patience, generosity, open-mindedness, punctuality and so on.

Contemplation

To round off the exercise, carry out the following Contemplation. Contemplation is heart thinking that penetrates our thoughts with feelings, passion and intentions. Contemplation is like an inner conversation with ourselves, in which we explore the meaning of our thoughts, values and core skills. As we contemplate, we make strong commitments to our thoughts, values and core skills in order to make them a part of our personality and daily life. As we contemplate our core skills, they become full of meaning and power. Contemplation has an energizing effect and charges our affirmations, making them a lot more effective.

Empty your consciousness and create an inner space of focused alertness by concentrating on your breathing only (Balanced Breathing). If concepts, memories or images appear, look at them calmly and then let them go (approx three minutes). Maintain the same breathing process throughout, to the end of the exercise.

Contemplate (heart thinking) the following core skills: calmness and security; caring and appreciation; strength and confidence; balance and harmony.

Contemplate images relating to sunlight. The following is an example of ways to contemplate the relationship between the symbol of the sun and our human consciousness and body:

The sun is the source of light, warmth and life, which correlate with the human virtues of wisdom (light), love (warmth) and strength (life). As the centre of the planetary system, the sun brings order to the planets in the same way that the human self brings order into the forces of consciousness. This order symbolizes the balance and harmony between cognition (wisdom), feeling (love) and will (strength); as our self creates this balance and harmony through personal development, the sun of the human spirit shines into the soul, experienced in our imagination as the sun shining within the human heart.

If you want to work on other core skills and qualities too, it is important to contemplate on them as well.

This Contemplation can be conducted as an inner conversation. For example, you can consider how your life will change as you acquire the skills and qualities you are contemplating.

Create strong feelings and intentions for these core skills. As you create those feelings and intentions in your Contemplation they will stay connected with these core values at other times as well, and will strengthen the effect of your affirmations and your mental rehearsal (see below).

The activity of Contemplation generally has a very energizing and vitalizing effect, when performed for approximately five minutes or longer.

Mental Rehearsing

Mental Rehearsing is an imagination technique. Mentally rehearsing core heart skills through your guided imagination is a powerful tool to help you manifest these new skills in your daily life.

Mentally rehearse applying your new skills (calmness, caring, confidence, harmony, and so on) in daily life by using the power of your imagination. To master the daily challenges of life more creatively and without events impacting on you negatively, picture yourself equipped with these core heart qualities, whether at home or at work.

Imagine reacting and acting out of those core heart qualities. Picture yourself mastering the challenges of life whilst feeling calm and secure, loving and appreciative, strong and confident. Picture yourself within your body, mastering any challenging situation with the creative power of your heart's intuitive intelligence.

Engage as many senses in this process as possible, such as smell, taste, touch, hearing, and make the image bright, large, loud (if not mentally rehearsing calmness) and sharp in focus. Activate the feelings attached to these images and core values, making them as strong as possible.

Picture, as vividly as possible, what your life will look like when you have acquired these core skills and apply them daily to yourself and others. As you picture your future as if it is happening now, feel the calmness, appreciation and confidence you generate with these images.

It is important not only to visualize (sensualize) the positive outcome of your endeavour and its consequences, but also the whole process or activity (rehearsing). The latter enhances performance and is skill building.

Ending the exercise

~ Experience gratitude and joy about the feelings you have received through your exercise.

~ Then slowly allow yourself to close the meditation. Imagine how you will return to the reality of daily life feeling refreshed and alert.

~ Stretch your whole body. Sit up, if you were lying down. Open your eyes.

Affirmation guidelines

~ Use 'you' and 'I' statements: this prompts your subconscious will to take the statements personally. ('You' = inhalation = hearing; 'I' = exhalation = speaking.)

~ Always state the phrase positively.

~ Stay in the present tense as if your desired goal is an accomplished fact: Say: 'I am calm, loving and strong' instead of 'I will be ...'

~ Focus predominantly on the sound of the words rather than on the content during the meditation.

~ Penetrate the content with conviction and intention.

~ Focus on the feelings and intentions associated with the affirmations. The feelings and intentions associated with your affirmations as well as your Mental Rehearsing can be greatly enhanced through Contemplation on your core skills. The process of Contemplation will make your affirmations and imaginations very powerful.

~ Repeat the affirmation rhythmically. Inwardly 'hear' the words being spoken to you as you inhale, and 'speak' the words as you exhale. 'Speak' the words quietly within, changing the inner volume from loud to whisper and then start loud again. Or imagine the words being spoken to you.

Struggling with the Heart Breathing exercise

For many people practising whole-chest breathing may initially be difficult.

The diaphragm may feel rigid and resistant, the breathing may stay shallow or become laboured.

Long-term exposure to stress and anxiety may have made relaxed breathing difficult.

If you should experience difficulties with the whole chest and abdominal breathing, a short preparatory breathing technique can be of help. The following exercise focusses on the exhalation in order to prepare yourself for deep, natural inhalation:

~ Inhale and exhale through your nose. Inhaling and exhaling through the nose creates a stronger resistance for the exhaled stream of air, and slows the breathing down and makes it deeper (diaphragmatic), without hyperventilating.

~ As you exhale, extend your exhalation, until it becomes approximately twice as long as your inhalation.

~ Exhale completely and wait until you feel the urge to inhale again.

~ Repeat this for three to seven breathing cycles.

~ You may feel an instant relaxation as you proceed and your breathing will naturally deepen as a result.

~ After 3–7 breathing cycles, you should move on to the Heart Breathing exercise as described above (whole chest and abdominal breathing, inhaling and exhaling through the nose, inhalation and exhalation equally long). This preparatory breathing technique can be very effective; it helps to enhance the exhalation process and prepares a relaxed breathing pattern. Nevertheless it should only be applied if necessary and if the experience is helpful.

Practise balanced breathing (without any affirmation or visualization) for short periods of time, as often as possible throughout the day, until this rhythm of breathing feels natural and easy to you.

Struggling with focus and concentration

During our meditation we can experience two tendencies:

~ We are *unable to relax* and are overwhelmed by thoughts and memories related to our daily life experience.

~ We *fall asleep* or enter into a state of dreaminess, being flooded with imagery.

Both tendencies take us away from our heart consciousness; they can appear in short succession. In order to maintain a balance between focus and relaxation, we have to maintain focus on our heart, which helps us to stay awake in, and in control within, our meditative consciousness. The following imagination may help to maintain this balance between sleep (dream and unconsciousness) and intellectual day consciousness:

~ Rather than imagining a contracting and expanding sphere of light as described above, as you inhale picture two beams of sunlight: one radiating down from the sky through your skull into your heart; the second beam radiating up from the centre of the earth through the base of your spine into your heart. Then imagine both beams uniting.

~ As you exhale, picture the two beams radiating out from the heart, one through the skull into the sky and the other through the base of the spine back to the centre of the earth.

~ Start imagining the movement of the upper beam first, and after several breathing cycles, imagine the movement of the lower beam only. In a third step imagine both beams simultaneously as they unite within your heart when you inhale and radiate out from your heart when you exhale.

~ Practise the same process with beams of sunlight from left and right and front and back, before uniting all these beams from opposite directions in the imagination of a pulsating sphere of light, breathing light in and out of body and heart from all directions simultaneously.

~ As you breathe the sunlight in and out, focus on the
   feelings of calmness, caring and confidence.

At the end of the exercise, Contemplation and Mental Rehearsing
should be done as has been described above. Imagining these
beams of light instead of the spheres of light is easier to master,
and you may find it significantly easier to achieve the optimal
balance between focus and relaxation.

Case Study: Overcoming Misery

~

In 2004 a lifetime of negative feelings — principally of anxiety
— were precipitated by family circumstances into a much more
acute depression with symptoms of sleeplessness, bursts of anger,
feelings of a failed and guilty life and suicidal imaginings.

Now, a year later, my life is transformed and I have a much
more balanced view of life in all its aspects. In Freud's phrase
(though not with his treatment methods) hysterical misery
has been replaced by ordinary unhappiness. This residual
unhappiness — which is mild rather than severe and does have
occasional sunny intervals — is I think attributable to a life-
long pre-disposition to unhappiness springing from childhood
and a failure to find ongoing creative activities.

Treatment at my medical practice has consisted of modest
doses of anti-depressant, now gradually being taken off, together
with regular coaching from Dr Gruenewald in HeartSpheres
techniques. These have consisted of the Heart Breathing
exercise, a combination of relaxation and breathing exercises
and affirmation.

In this process I have developed, with Dr Gruenewald's
flexible approach to treatment, a series of helpful mental
pictures (the essence of which came to me unbidden). In these

I see a series of coloured veils fall from a 'diamond' version of myself, to be replaced by more luminously coloured positive feelings within the transparent self that arises, phoenix-like, from each negative veil consumed by the fire of love. Each major negative feeling is replaced by an inwardly and outwardly directed positive feeling.

A red veil of anger is replaced by patience and loving kindness.

A yellow veil of fear is replaced by courage and trust.

A green veil of envy is replaced by gratitude and empathy.

A white veil of perfectionism is replaced by self-forgiveness and an ability to enjoy the unexpected.

After stopping the anti-depressant treatment I see myself continuing HeartSpheres-based exercises and also continuing with new creative activities and making other lifestyle changes as may be necessary.

My treatment has provided a foundation for this future of balanced thinking and feeling.

L.T., architect, aged 62

Contemplation (positive self-talk)

Our daily life experience is constantly accompanied by our inner voice talking silently to us. This self-talk judges circumstances and situations, both those of ourselves and of others. It thus helps us to process the past, to cope with events happening in the present and to manage future events. Comments, judgements and assumptions such as, 'If only ...'; 'How bad ...'; 'How wonderful ...'; 'I will never be able to manage ...'; 'This is easy, I can do that ...' are expressions of our own beliefs and values based on past experience, personality, character and feelings. They reflect our current emotional state and also determine how we respond to immediate and future events.

Our own inner voice mostly runs on autopilot. It is there, whether we want it or not. As negative self-talk, this inner voice can exaggerate problems, deepen despair, 'catastrophize' experiences, undermine our trust in ourselves and others through excessive criticism, devaluing others and undervaluing ourselves.

Or, as illusionary self-talk, it can create unrealistic judgements about ourselves and others. We may then overestimate our skills and underestimate risks and/or the seriousness of situations.

In both cases this inner voice reflects our emotional state on the spectrum between exaggerating euphoria, excessive joy and recklessness on the one hand, and paralysing sadness, despair, fear and anxiety on the other.

Because our emotional state and inner voice influence our judgement and decision-making, ultimately they affect our actions too.

As we learn to take charge of our inner voice and begin to guide it consciously, we find ways of managing our emotional state. Instead of running our lives in 'autopilot mode', we can learn to master this inner voice, master our inner emotional state and ultimately our lives. Often we may not be able to change our outer circumstances immediately, but we can change our inner response to them and this can make all the difference.

Contemplation, or heart thinking, is an inner voice that integrates and unites thoughts, feelings and intentions and places them under the sway of our higher self. In Contemplation we can use our inner voice to explore life questions. Likewise we can use it to examine, form and develop values and beliefs about ourselves and others. Through Contemplation we can transform the way we respond emotionally to events, we can learn to create powerful tools to enhance insights, and to create strong motives for our actions.

Contemplation helps develop a golden mean between emotional extremes, enhancing enthusiasm, true appreciation, love and compassion. This heart-based, balanced, inner conversation with ourselves always starts with an existential question, such as:

~ How do I deal with this life issue confronting me?

~ Who am I?

~ What are my weaknesses and strengths?

~ How can I change and develop?

~ What are the obstacles to my development?

~ How do I want my life to look in 1, 2, 5, 10 or 20 years?

~ Why am I still in my job?

~ How can I transform a destructive relationship into one that can further the development of all involved?

We can explore the answers to any one of these questions through an inner conversation with ourselves that is based on a synthesis of thinking, feeling and intentions. Such a self-guided inner exploration is usually found to be life-enhancing and energizing. It avoids emotional extremes and firmly roots itself in a deep appreciation for ourselves, others and life as a whole. Developing from one of the existential questions above, we can go on to ask more universal questions:

~ What do I truly appreciate about myself, others and life as a whole?

~ How can I see my and other people's current problems as part of our personal development?

~ How can I understand the present situation as dictated by the past?

~ What future potential lies within this situation?

Without turning a blind eye to the difficulties and problems, but also without indulging in destructive criticism, this golden middle path of Contemplation connects with our emotional intelligence, developing intuitive insights into ourselves and others, resolving conflicts and creating strong motives for our actions.

As we practise deep, Balanced Breathing during active Contemplation, we support mental activity by maintaining our physiological equilibrium.

The following four exercises apply Contemplation:

a. Problem Solving
b. Accessing Core Values
c. Developing Appreciation
e. Inner Dialogue

Problem Solving

The Problem Solving exercise is a powerful tool to open and access the creativity of your mind so as to address daily problems effectively.

It will enable you to distance yourself from the negativity attached to the problem and to develop a confident, positive attitude, so that you start to see the related issues in a wider and less self-centred context.

~ Focus on a problem that has been affecting you.

~ Write down anything that relates to your problem: all your thoughts, feelings and intentions.

~ Now put aside what you have written.

~ Shift your focus away from your problem: close your eyes and focus on someone or something you truly appreciate. As you develop thoughts and feelings of appreciation or gratitude, practise Balanced Breathing as described earlier. This can be done for 2 to 5 minutes.

~ Now open your eyes. Turn the paper around and write down all your thoughts, feelings and intentions related to your problem, without reading what you had written before.

~ When you have completed your task, look back and find out whether you think, feel and intend acting differently now. What has changed? You may be surprised…

Accessing Core Values

> A person will worship something, have no doubt about
> that. We may think our tribute is paid in secret in the
> dark recesses of our hearts, but it will out. That which
> dominates our imaginations and our thoughts will
> determine our lives, and our character. Therefore, it
> behoves us to be careful what we worship, for what we
> are worshipping we are becoming.

Ralph Waldo Emerson (1803–82)

Creating motives for our actions

Rarely do we find ourselves fully aware of the driving forces
behind our actions. Much of what we do is ruled by our physiological needs, such as hunger and sex drive, and also environmen-
tal influences such as culture, social class and family. Becoming
aware of our personal needs, core values and aspirations, as well
as the obstacles to fulfilling them, is a first step towards bringing
creativity and self-determination into our lives.

In our contemplative thinking we can create motives for
our actions, such as sincerity and compassion. Through our
creative thinking we can develop ideas about how we want to
live our lives in future. When contemplating core values and
aspirations within the specific context of our life, we can harmonize, order and prioritize them. By becoming aware of our
motives and learning to develop them through contemplative
thinking, we 'invite them in' so that they increasingly influence our actions.

We can transform these motives (intuitions) into practi-
cal ideals by imbuing them with passion and enthusiasm.
(See Inner Dialogue p.51, and Transforming Disturbing
Emotions, p.85.)

Only when we transform our ideals into specific and tangible imaginative pictures, creating a vision of future reality, can we engage with and shape our future reality and actions. We can achieve this when we engage in active imagination or sensualization. (See Mental Rehearsing, p.75.)

On the other hand, over-attachment and over-identification need to be recognized and transformed, as do emotional distance or lack of attachment. The best way to find out what or who we are over-attached to is by asking whether being with this person or dealing with this issue drains or increases our energy. Extreme emotions can drain our energy levels and leave us tired and exhausted. This can be linked with excessively high expectations of ourselves and others, and fantasies about worst-case scenarios — which in turn can increase anxieties and the fear of failure, anger, frustration and so on.

Lack of attachment and identification (for instance, 'stonewalling,' cool detachment, indifference and so on) can be the result of deep-seated feelings of anger, resentment, frustration, fear, guilt and hatred, which we may not be aware of. Lack of interest and boredom in an encounter with another person or towards professional activities, for example, can be very problematic too. These attitudes may not immediately be disturbing for us, but can be the cause of major stress in others and will therefore negatively impact on our lives as well.

After recognizing and experiencing the disturbing feelings associated with our over- or under-attachments and over- and under-identifications, we can reduce and neutralize their impact by developing inner calm and security. Inner self-talk can help us transform issues of attachment and identification into caring and compassion for ourselves and others and into passion for the areas of life that are important to us. In so doing, we can overcome the energy drain of extreme emotions, creating new energy, passion and constructive commitment. (See Inner Dialogue, p.51.)

One of the prerequisites for this is to recognize issues of attachment and identification, and the feelings, thoughts and actions attached to them. By identifying areas of concern you learn to relate to them in a different way. You need to know your motives and aspirations, and the obstacles and steps towards their realization, in order to make progress.

The Core Values worksheet (see below) can help you to become aware of the aspirations and life objectives you care most about, and understand how they impact on you. It will help you to become more aware of the direction in which you steer your exercises and, ultimately, your life. In completing the questionnaire, you will contemplate major life issues affecting you and may have to come to terms with some strong emotions too. It is therefore advisable to start with a few cycles of Balanced Breathing and the activation of feeling of calmness, appreciation and confidence.

Begin with the first column in Part A of the Core Values Worksheet. Select four areas of life where you have issues, which are most important to you and note them down in Column 1. These issues don't need to be noted down in any particular sequence, as you will be able to grade their level of importance in Column 2 and so prioritize them. In Column 3 note your thoughts, feelings and actions related to the areas you have identified. Now move on to Columns 4 and 5, where you should describe what achieving or not achieving your aspirations related to these issues would mean for you. In Column 6 write down what obstacles you have or may encounter on the path of realizing your aspirations. Finally, answer the three questions in Part B regarding beliefs about yourself and circumstances that either support or inhibit you.

After completing the worksheet, put it away; then pick it up again after a few days and go through it carefully. This will help you to select the areas you may want to work on using the Inner Dialogue and Mental Rehearsing exercises.

Two examples are built into the questionnaire that follows.

Core Values Worksheet

Core Values Worksheet: Part A (see opposite) and Part B (see below)

What supportive and encouraging beliefs do you hold about yourself? (I can / I am)	*Example* I am able to change. I can make a difference.
What inhibiting and discouraging beliefs do you hold about yourself? (I can't, etc.)	*Example* At times I feel hopeless and defeated. I believe that I deserve things to turn against me at times. I believe that I only deserve to be loved, if I live up to my or other people's expectations.
What circumstances strengthen your determination and perseverance?	*Example* Praise. Success. Being appreciated.

What are the issues that matter most to you in your life?	Grading (1–5 where 5 = very important)	What do you feel about them?	What would you like to do about these issues?	What would be the result if you can't resolve them?	What stops you from resolving them?
My mother lives by herself. She has aged fast, has become forgetful and had a couple of falls. I am living 150 miles away from her and can visit her only rarely. I would like to see her safe and well cared for.	5	I feel worried and guilty that I cannot look after her. I am worried that she may not cope on her own. I ring her every day to find out whether she is well. I visit her about once every six weeks. I discuss the issues with my husband and my siblings.	I would feel very relieved, if I knew that mother was safe and well cared for.	I would feel guilty, worried and burdened. Being stressed about my mother may take a toll on my life with my husband and my children.	Distance, not having access to support agencies and her local doctor.
Being calmer, more laid back, less irritable, less angry. I wish I could be more calm and composed in challenging situations	5	I have caused a lot of upset around me due to bouts of anger and irritability. I feel unhappy that I am so little in control of my reactions.	It would help me to develop a better relationship with my wife and children.	It puts my relationship with my wife and children at risk. I may be at risk of a heart attack due to stress, grief and unresolved anger.	I can't do it without help. I am sometimes not in charge of my emotional response and how I react. I haven't tried systematic exercises or counselling yet.

Developing Appreciation

Close your eyes and practise the Heart Breathing exercise, focusing on the feeling of appreciation and its affirmation. Then drop visualization (sunlight and heart) as well as the affirmation, maintaining only Balanced Breathing and the feeling of appreciation.

Now start exploring yourself and others by taking the first step in formulating a question. Some examples follow on p.50:

Exploring myself:

~ What do I truly appreciate about myself? (Developing appreciation.)

~ How do I understand my own difficulties or weaknesses in the light of my past experiences? (Developing understanding and compassion for myself.)

~ What is my future developmental potential — what may I achieve by transforming difficulties or weaknesses into progress, skills and virtues? (Developing confidence and determination.)

~ What do I want to achieve in life? What are the next steps in my personal and professional development? (Developing goals.)

~ What are the obstacles to such development?

~ What skills do I need to acquire and what help do I need to seek out in order to overcome obstacles to positive development?

~ How do I want to do this — what are the steps I need
  to take? (Developing strategies.)

As you explore these questions in your inner conversation,
maintain Balanced Breathing and the feeling of appreciation
for yourself and others.

This process should be regularly repeated, at least once a
week if possible, exploring the same area of life repeatedly or
moving on from one area to the next.

As you slowly increase your capacity not only to explore
problems but also to open yourself to solutions, mentally
rehearse the skills required at the end of the exercise (see
Mental Rehearsing). This will help you develop vision for your
future. As you develop vision, your ideas from the realm of
thinking (idea) and feeling (enthusiasm) will begin to penetrate
the realm of will (action). You will be prepared to act upon the
values, motives and intention that you have created in the above
process (skills), carrying them into reality (deeds).

Exploring others:
Practise the same activity, as described above, but focusing now
on the other person. The same questions apply as when exploring yourself.

Stop short, though, of practising Mental Rehearsing for others,
as this part of the exercise should only be applied to yourself.

We can develop understanding, compassion and trust in the
other person, but it is better to leave the initiative for overcoming difficulties to them, unless they ask us to help.

Inner Dialogue

The Inner Dialogue exercise helps to develop a deep sense
of appreciation for ourselves and others. Difficult social relationships can be fundamentally changed by processing and

transforming negative emotions and attitudes, enabling us to connect empathetically with other people or ourselves. We can learn to recognize the impact which negative or traumatic experiences and challenging relationships have on our daily life and health. We also learn how to alleviate the impact of these traumatic experiences. We can transform our attitudes and emotional responses by tapping into our own and other people's developmental potential for positive change.

This exercise teaches us to overcome limiting fear, anxiety, grief, anger and frustration. It teaches us to transform criticism and negativity into appreciation, compassion and forgiveness.

The Inner Dialogue is a Contemplation exercise that works like an inner conversation with ourselves. As we experience the strains of work, confrontation with work colleagues, tension between family members, the joys of socializing with friends or family, and any other daily life experiences, we tend to comment on our own behaviour and personality in a critical or approving manner. We do this in the form of an inner conversation with ourselves. This inner conversation usually happens without us controlling the direction and content of this dialogue. Our criticism and approval are then just a reflection of our self-image and our attitudes towards others. The emotional response triggered by a daily event is strongly influenced by our past experiences.

We can learn to master the Inner Dialogue and give it our own direction and content. We can re-live past experiences and human encounters and re-process their emotional content by developing equanimity, insight, appreciation, compassion and forgiveness towards ourselves and others. As we practise the Inner Dialogue within a relaxed, but focused imaginative state of mind, it will help us to transform ourselves and improve our relationships.

Developing appreciation, understanding, compassion, acceptance and forgiveness for yourself and others rather than guilt feelings, or being excessively self-critical or critical, will help you overcome major obstacles to your personal development and will open the doors for transforming yourself and your life. This in turn will strengthen your ability to take responsibility for your actions and for your destiny.

Self-destructive criticism and guilt feelings are as much an obstacle to personal development as is the turning of a blind eye to our own weaknesses and blaming others for our misfortunes.

Our personality traits and our destiny can only be transformed in depth, if we first acknowledge, accept and forgive the weaknesses and problems of ourselves and others. Compassion is a powerful path towards acceptance and forgiveness. Without deep and sincere forgiveness for ourselves and others we are likely to stay trapped in the effects of past experiences on our personality, and remain unable to take full responsibility for ourselves and our destiny.

The Inner Dialogue exercise is divided into five main parts, which build upon each other, in order to help you focus on each process with sufficient intensity.

It is best to read the instructions for this exercise carefully a few times. Try to remember the different parts of the exercise, perhaps even noting them down for yourself in your own words.

The main parts of the Inner Dialogue exercise are:

a. Focused relaxation (Heart Breathing exercise)
b. Identifying and describing the facts of the current situation
c. Focusing on yourself
d. Focusing on the other person or event
e. Developing genuine appreciation for yourself and others

A. *Focused relaxation*

Enter into a state of focused relaxation with a short Heart Breathing exercise, using the affirmation of calmness, caring and confidence (balance). The focused and relaxed state will allow the effect of the Inner Dialogue exercise to powerfully expand into transforming your subconscious, changing your emotional responses and actions. Maintain Balanced Breathing throughout the whole Inner Dialogue exercise. (See Heart Breathing exercise, p.25.)

B. *Identify and describe the facts of the current situation*

Now focus on a difficult relationship or a difficult event.

Describe the actual facts of the event. What has really happened? Try to avoid any judgements about yourself or the other person(s) and just focus on the actual event. This may initially be difficult, as we are used to entangling judgements with our perceptions without even being aware of it.

Observe and describe the facts of a situation without immediate personal judgement. As judgements about yourself and others tends to appear within your mind, try to hold them back in order to delay them. Looking at a situation by delaying judgement will allow you to view this situation in a deeper and more profound way, and to develop intuitive insight. (See Intuitive Conversation, p.81, and Extending Sensory Perceptions, p.91.)

C. *Focus on yourself*

Experience, ease and understand negative emotions or behaviours associated with difficult social relationships and/or traumatic events.

~ Continue to *breathe* slowly, regularly and with your whole chest and abdomen throughout the entire exercise.

~ *Experience* the feelings attached to a person, situation or to yourself. What were my feelings at the time, what was my emotional and behavioural response? Was I angry, frustrated, anxious, fearful or upset? Or was I inappropriately detached and cold?

~ *Ease* these feelings where necessary by developing and maintaining inner calmness. Picturing yourself from outside (in the distance) can help to ease these feelings. Imagine that you breathe in calmness and security, which penetrate and ease your feelings of fear, anxiety, anger, grief etc. without suppressing them.

~ Or *amplify* the feelings connected with this situation if they appear too weak or detached. You can amplify the feelings by picturing the event, whilst experiencing it from inside your body.

~ *Understand* your negative feelings or problematic response without criticizing yourself or feeling guilty.

~ Try to understand how these feelings and emotional responses have arisen from your own unmet needs in that particular situation and in the past. Understand what impact your emotional response may have on yourself and on the other person? (Why did/does this person affect me so strongly? Which of my needs were not met?)

Transform negative emotions through acceptance, compassion and forgiveness for yourself:

~ Develop thoughts and feelings of *compassion* for yourself.

~ You can picture yourself as a young child being deeply hurt by the event. As you develop a deep sense of compassion for this *'hurt inner child,'* you can extend this compassion to yourself and your current life situation.

~ Experience how compassion *dissolves disturbing emotions* attached to yourself, objects or a situation you are contemplating.

~ Develop a sense of *acceptance and/or forgiveness* for yourself. Take enough time to go through this step fully.

~ Take *responsibility* for yourself and others and particularly for your feelings, actions and your destiny.

Mentally rehearse personal and social skills:

~ Imagine that you are endowed with calmness, caring, confidence and harmony, and/or other core qualities.

~ Consider how you may be able to contribute to resolving the conflict or the difficulties. Ask your heart and feelings what the most appropriate action is on your part.

~ Picture how you solve the problems in your own and the other person's best interest.

~ Picture yourself perceiving and expressing your own, and the other person's feelings, needs and requests with empathy, and without criticizing, expecting or demanding anything. (Picture yourself within your body.)

~ Develop a sense of joy, caring and appreciation about this way of dealing with the situation. (See Mental Rehearsing, p.75.)

Working on your own emotional and behavioural responses first helps develop the necessary insight into your own personality, giving self-knowledge and the courage and trust in yourself to take responsibility for your own life. This will help you to be less judgemental and more insightful about yourself before moving on to understanding the other person.

D.   Focus on the other person involved

Having done the previous steps of describing the facts and recognizing and transforming our own attitudes, emotions and behavioural responses, we are now ready to work on a deeper understanding and acceptance of the other person.

Identify the feelings, needs and motives of the other person involved in this situation:

~ How did the person act or express himself or herself at the time?

~ What were the person's feelings at the time?

~ Which of their needs were not met in the situation?

~ What requests did the person make?

~ Avoid criticism. Instead develop a deep interest for the feelings and unmet needs of the other person.

Develop a deep sense of compassion, acceptance and forgiveness for the other person:

~ Develop thoughts and feelings of compassion.

~ Feel how compassion for that other person dissolves the disturbing emotions triggered in you by the other person or situation. (You may relate to the 'hurt, inner child' within the other person as you develop your compassion.)

~ Develop a sense of acceptance and/or forgiveness for the other person.

Ask your heart how to best resolve your conflict or difficulties, so that both of you may benefit from the relationship:

~ Consider how you may be able to contribute to resolving your conflict.

~ Ask your heart what the most appropriate action is on your part.

E. Developing genuine appreciation for yourself and others

~ Reflect on your own positive qualities and/or those of a friend, relative, colleague or neighbour. Don't just list these qualities, but ponder on the impact they have on your or the other person's life and social environment.

~ Develop a deep sense of appreciation of these qualities. Focus on thoughts and feelings of appreciation.

~ End this exercise by sending feelings of calmness, caring and strength towards yourself and others. You can support this activity with the affirmation: 'May calmness, caring and strength live within us.'

Comment:

Initially it is important to apply this exercise to relationships and situations which are not too troublesome or traumatic. As you progress with the exercise, you can start working on more difficult relationships and situations. It can also be very helpful to process past relationships and events, for example childhood experiences, in order to transform the impact they have on your current life. Furthermore you can address and transform deep-seated personality traits by accepting them with compassion and forgiveness and mentally rehearsing new skills within your imagination. You may find it difficult to ease the feelings that surface, and find yourself overwhelmed by them. Should this happen, neutralize the negative emotional associations these events have triggered by practising emotional detachment with the help of Day Review (reframing past experiences), on p.68.

Case Study: Living with a Demanding Mother

~

I am 43 years old, married with three children (now aged 13, 15 and 3). I work as an electronics engineer, developing and designing products for computers.

My mother has been living with the family for the past four years. This decision was based on a certain necessity but also on genuine mutual fondness. The first two years went well and everybody was pleased with the arrangement. This has changed dramatically over the past two years.

When I first saw Dr Gruenewald, I felt emotionally drained and physically exhausted. I felt that my enjoyment in life had been lost. What kept me going was my sense of duty towards my family. I felt that I was just going through the motions of life, although I was not sure whether there was much point in that at all.

I didn't want to end my life, but I would have liked to just fall asleep and not wake up. I had stopped enjoying activities I previously enjoyed, for example socializing with friends. I believed that the cause of all my problems was the drastic change in the relationship with my mother.

My mother had become increasingly demanding: constantly complaining, and interfering with our family life. She was insensitive to everyone else's needs, and intrusive.

I blamed myself for the fact that my wife and family found life with my mother (and with me!) increasingly difficult. The only one who still liked having his grandmother around was my three-year-old son, who has a sunny disposition and seems happy anywhere.

Over the last few months I had become irritable, often very angry and short-tempered, full of guilt and confusion about my own behaviour. I avoided my mother wherever I could, as a measure of self-protection.

I had been feeling very resentful towards her, partly because I started to remember a lot of negative experiences from the past and because I blamed her for all our current problems.

She did not show any understanding for my very busy and demanding work, nor the circumstances of my wife or teenage children. I felt trapped, and could not see a way out. I also felt depressed and developed other health problems.

I found it difficult to speak to my friends about the home situation because I thought that all my problems might sound petty and ridiculous. I felt ashamed and worried that they might consider me as a complete failure and unable to deal with my problems adequately.

All this has impacted not only on my relationship with my wife and children, but also on my work, and it was this which finally drove me to consult a doctor.

I had developed sleep problems, high blood pressure, and frequent headaches, and I kept worrying about my more or less constant, dull stomach ache.

Dr Gruenewald took himself time to listen to me and asked me to come again for a thirty minute appointment. He arranged for some medical investigations (blood test), which besides increased cholesterol and slightly raised blood pressure all turned out to be normal.

At the second consultation Dr Gruenewald invited me to see him for a one-to-one coaching session of the HeartSpheres approach. He suggested teaching me techniques which would empower me to cope better with my life situation and social relationships and that could help to improve my low mood.

I was motivated to give it a go as I saw a possibility of avoiding medication and counselling, which I had not been so keen on anyway.

Dr Gruenewald suggested that counselling or medication may still be needed, but agreed to pursue the HeartSpheres approach first.

In my first session Dr Gruenewald gave me an overview of the HeartSpheres approach and its clinical background. He introduced the Balanced Breathing technique to me, and suggested that I should practise it at least once daily for ten minutes, but more frequently, if possible.

In my session seven days later he introduced the rest of the Heart Breathing exercise, but suggested initially practising the affirmation of calmness and security for a few days and than slowly adding the other parts when I felt confident to do so.

He advised me to practise the Heart Breathing exercise once or twice daily for ten to thirty minutes. Within a few days of practising the Heart Breathing exercise I experienced a new sense of inner calmness not only during the exercise but as well, at least at times, throughout the day.

After about two weeks I realized that I had been significantly more relaxed in the communication with all members of my family, including my mother. My wife confirmed that change.

I started to feel less anxious and irritable and became able to stay calm in many of the challenging situations. I had been practising about twice a day for at least fifteen minutes, and had enjoyed it and considered it as my personal quality time. As soon as I practised controlled regular breathing, I experienced a deep sense of calmness and relaxation.

My low mood had not much improved though; when I saw Dr Gruenewald again two weeks after the previous consultation, I was still feeling low most of the time. But I felt encouraged by the progress I had made with my fears and irritability and I felt generally more hopeful..

During this session Dr Gruenewald introduced the Inner Dialogue exercises. He advised me to spend only up to twenty minutes on the Heart Breathing exercise and then to move on to the Inner Dialogue exercise.

Practising the Inner Dialogue exercise I started to recollect very recent situations. In the evening I looked back to encounters with my mother during the day. I tried to remember each situation as vividly as possible. I tried to visualize my mother's and my own gestures, facial expressions, spoken and unspoken words, and how I felt in the situation.

I learned how to cope with my feelings attached to the memories by continuing with Balanced Breathing and feeling deep calmness.

The feelings I experienced at the time were anger, annoyance, frustration and sadness. I learned how to ease these feelings and how to look at the situation in a more detached way. Moving on to the next step of the exercise I learned to develop feelings of compassion for myself, something I have never done before in my life. The image of the hurt child within me was a great help. I then moved on to mentally rehearsing difficult life situations by picturing myself in difficult situations with my mother and finding calmness, caring and strength to resolve these situations amicably.

Having practised this for a while, I started to apply this exercise to my mother. I reflected on some of the personal traits in her which I really appreciate, and allowed myself to create and experience feelings of appreciation for her. For example I admire her patience in dealing with my children.

In a next step I faced the difficult aspects of our relationship, not criticizing now, but rather trying to understand her behaviour and reactions from her perspective and by reflecting upon her own difficult childhood experiences.

From here it was not too difficult any more to develop a sense of compassion for my mother as I recognized how little she seemed to be in charge of her behaviour and her own emotional responses. As I experienced compassion for her and her current life situation, I extended this compassion to her 'victims' too (that is, my family and myself). I ended the exercise by asking myself, how to best respond to this life situation in order to find a solution to the conflict.

I practised this exercise about four times and experienced a significant change within myself after a few days.

I learned to develop a sense of acceptance not only for her, but for my failures too. I learned to see our whole situation in a different light.

The change of attitude towards myself and my mother changed my perspective on our problems, and I can respond to her better, even in challenging daily situations.

For example I can feel my mother's pain and concern and understand the motives for her actions.

I gradually have come to recognize that she has no intention to harm anyone.

Also, surprisingly, it has not been too difficult to replace blaming my mother, other family members or myself with positive assertiveness, understanding and forgiveness. Of course this works better on some days than on others, but I have realized that there are issues which need more work and others which now seem to be resolving almost effortlessly.

What surprised me most was that although I had never talked to my mother about the exercises I had been doing, she seemed to have been changing too, opening up and showing more interest in the family's life again.

The relationship with my family has improved as well and I feel optimistic about the future.

The physical symptoms have eased up, in step with the disappearing tension.

I have made the Heart Breathing exercise and the Inner Dialogue exercise a regular part of my life now. I have learned to use and adapts them to my own needs for other situations, for example for difficult relationships at work. I do seem to get on a lot better with family, friends and colleagues.

B.R., 43 years, engineer

Case Study: From Carer to Companion

~

Celia S., a carer for children with special needs, describes her experience with the Inner Dialogue exercise as follows:

I have been working for about 8 months with a twelve-year-old girl, Angela, with moderate learning difficulties and autistic spectrum disorder. Most people find it hard to communicate with her at all, so I am grateful that I have been able to build up some kind of relationship.

I have the feeling Angela has developed some trust in me.

What makes life difficult for Angela is her unpredictability, often combined with outbursts and violent actions, such as screeching, throwing objects and pulling hair. It is sad to see her life reduced to a very restricted environment and also to see people withdraw from her out of fear, especially as her aggression is rarely aimed at people directly.

After having worked with Angela for about four months I realized that I needed to develop more understanding for her, to be able to intervene in or even prevent these outbursts, and to enable her to have a more fulfilled life.

I came across the Inner Dialogue exercise through a friend and decided to give it a go.

I had realized before that there was no direct route to exert some kind of control over Angela's destructive behaviour. Rather than manipulating I would have liked to empower her to be more in control of herself.

I knew from her parents, the carers before me and also from my experience that nobody could control Angela, even if they wanted to. Somehow we became reduced to clearing dangerous stuff out of her way, trying to keep her content by second-guessing her needs and doing damage control, when the chairs or cutlery were flying ...

My frustration made me open to the way the Inner Dialogue exercise works. I started to build up a deep inner relationship to Angela by visualizing her outer appearance, then her movements, her language and facial expressions, and finally by reliving situations of her life. I tried to relive her experiences and actions. After a while I imagined that I could experience how she must have felt in those situations. I started with situations of conflict, because that seemed the obvious thing, but I then also started to try to picture her in ordinary daily life. After only a couple of weeks I realized that I could experience her pain and fear within me in ordinary life circumstances. All of a sudden Angela was not unpredictable any more. I could anticipate her outbursts, which usually were reactions to events in her environment that deeply scared her, or people who from her (and by now also my) point of experience invaded her private space, which terrified her.

We started to go into public spaces more frequently now, from shops to small musical performances or a gallery. Through the exercises I had not only learned to understand Angela's reactions better, but I had also developed a deep respect for how she dealt with her life. I think this allowed a transformation from my role as a carer, from functioning more or less as a guard to keep her and others safe and deal with unpleasant side effects, into a friend or companion.

I also realized that often I could not only anticipate her reactions, but appreciate them.

The really strange thing is that Angela seems to have a lot fewer outbursts than previously, not because of my anticipation and therefore 'rescuing' her from the situation, but because she seems to feel that I understand her and that makes her feel safe.

Her family has realized this too and I talked with them about the exercises. I am not sure whether they will ever do them too, but there has been a subtle change in their attitude towards Angela. They seem to experience and treat her more like a person and not as a loved, but slightly scary and very embarrassing phenomenon. This in turn seems to relax Angela, and their life together has changed for the better, because there is a lot less tension.

Celia J., 25 years, carer

Day Review (reframing past experiences)

Caution: Should you suffer from the effects of severe trauma then do not attempt to work on highly traumatic events without the help of a qualified therapist, as you may put yourself at risk of re-traumatization and aggravation of your symptoms.

> I don't avoid pain by not remembering something; I try to remember .... Memory is empowering, and it's what gives you your sense of continuity in the world.
>
> *Melinda Worth Popham*

Reframing is the process of reviewing the past event from the observer perspective (looking at yourself from outside). This exercise helps to neutralize the effect that past, possibly traumatic, experiences have on our emotions. As we learn to review the event by stepping out of our body and seeing ourselves from outside, as if in the far distance, we are able to neutralize the strong negative and often destructive emotions connected with this memory. This process is helped by maintaining emotional control through controlled, regular breathing. As we practise this exercise, disturbing emotions and memories will no longer overwhelm us when we are exposed to similar situations.

Recollecting and sensualizing* events of the day or the more distant past can teach us to develop calmness and a sense of security, which we can carry into challenging daily circumstances. This exercise creates inner objectivity and cultivates calmness, equanimity and intuitive insight with ourselves and others. The negative impact of past events on current and future life situations can be reduced and neutralized through the calmness and objectivity this exercise engenders.

---

* Visualization broadened to all the senses, such as hearing, taste, touch, and so on.

This exercise is best done before going to bed and can last approximately ten to twenty minutes.

Enter into a state of focused relaxation

~ Choose a quiet place and time, and sit in a comfortable position. Enter into a state of deep, focused relaxation with a short Heart Breathing exercise, practising the affirmation related to calmness and security.

~ Activate the feeling of calm detachment and try to sustain it throughout the exercise.

~ As you go into a state of focused relaxation, your subconscious mind is open to learning new ways of dealing with the challenge.

Review the event(s) (up to ten minutes)

~ Select an experience you had today. You can also apply this exercise to any past event. Initially this experience should not be emotionally loaded as it needs practice, and often personal guidance, to learn to deal with emotionally charged or traumatic experiences.

~ Review the event by looking at it and yourself, from outside. You become your own observer by seeing yourself from outside (dissociation). Initially you can step behind yourself, see yourself from behind and even from above. As you are able to stay emotionally detached you can start observing yourself from the front.

~ Picture the situation in as much detail as possible. Details you don't remember can be recreated imaginatively, in order to form a complete picture.

~ Stay calm and emotionally uninvolved.

~ Avoid any judgement or self-judgement during this exercise.

~ Roll the event backwards, that is, in reverse, from the end to the beginning. This will help you to avoid reflecting on the events too intellectually, and will engage your will more strongly and effectively in processing the event.

~ Staying outside yourself as observer throughout the exercise will prevent you from getting emotionally over-involved.

~ As you progress, you will be able to review most of the day's events within ten minutes.

Rounding off

~ Let go of all images and thoughts. Focus on the feeling of calmness and security created through this review exercise and try to sustain it for a period of time. If you get distracted by images, thoughts and feelings, look at them and then send them away and refocus on controlled breathing and the feeling of calmness.

~ Sustain the feelings of calmness and security.

~ End as in the Heart Breathing exercise.

Additional advice

At times it can be hard to maintain the dissociated observer consciousness whilst reviewing emotionally charged events. We may feel drawn back into our body, immediately experiencing distress, anger and upset, rather then developing a detached and calm relationship to the event. The depth of breathing may change under the influence of those emotions. This has to be avoided as it renders the exercise ineffective and can even be harmful as it can lead to re-traumatization.

In order to create a stronger distance between you as the observer and the event you can do the following:

~ Maintain distance by erecting a glass wall between yourself as the observer and you as the remembered and imagined person involved in the event. The glass wall will prevent your return into your body and maintains the distance required.

~ And/or you can project the event on to a cinema screen observing yourself and the situation you were involved in, as if in a movie.

~ Shrink the image, freeze it, silence it or make it black and white in order to reduce the impact this memory has on generating disturbing emotions.

~ Maintain Balanced Breathing and a feeling of calm detachment throughout the whole exercise.

Case Study: Frustration of a Teenager

~

I was in my A-level year and found it extremely stressful. I wanted to study law and needed very good results. I was always a good student but was at odds with my history teacher. I felt that he hated me and wanted me to fail, but was himself incompetent in some areas of the subject. We often used to have words, where I felt he was in the right, but my teacher just wouldn't admit it. He was out to get me!

I was so worked up and frustrated that it had a negative effect on my attitude to school. I became extremely bad-tempered and started falling out with my sister, who claims I had become unbearable. I felt that nobody understood the pressure I was under, blamed family and friends for not caring and talked about giving it all up and going travelling to get rid of them all. But I also felt ill all the time and wondered whether I had the strength for travelling on the cheap.

I decided to see Dr Gruenewald only as a (last) favour to my parents, and in the beginning I was not very engaged at all. I must have come across as impatient and arrogant. As our conversation continued, I felt safe to open up and poured out my grievances. After a while I even enjoyed the conversation, as I realized that I wasn't being criticized or blamed.

I agreed to start with some relaxation exercises to help me to calm down, because I somehow felt sad and frustrated that I kept losing my temper with the people I liked and cared about.

A week or two after practising the exercises almost daily, my sleep started to improve, even though I had not even realized before that my sleep quality had deteriorated over the last few months. I felt more relaxed and able to open up and engage in conversations.

Through my conversations with Dr Gruenewald I realized that I can become very impatient with people and that I have really high expectations of myself and others and hate to see them disappointed. I mentioned to him that I have often been perceived as arrogant and that I didn't think this was the case at all, but that people often misunderstood me.

I just like to get things right and find it extremely annoying if people who should be knowledgeable in certain areas do not get their facts straight. I found teachers particularly annoying because they had an automatic claim to always being right and never admitted to mistakes. I couldn't stand their hypocritical behaviour, 'demanding respect,' when they did not respect me at all. I just couldn't understand how this did not seem to matter to other people.

I felt, though, that I often got things a bit out of perspective and wished to be more patient and slower to judge others. I did not like the fact that I sometimes treated people, even friends, unfairly because of my quick temper.

I agreed to work on my relationship with the teacher after Dr Gruenewald introduced the Inner Dialogue exercise to me. I was keen to try this exercise, because I felt that this relationship had so much impact on my life at present and for the future, and I hoped that the exercise would help.

At times I had been extremely harsh in my judgement about myself and others. I understood that being kinder with myself and learning to accept my own weaknesses would help me to be kinder towards others.

After two weeks of practising the Inner Dialogue exercise I felt that my attitude towards my teacher had changed. At times I was now able to see the teacher's point of view. We still had disagreements, but they seemed to be more constructive. Sometimes it happened now that I could convince my teacher of my own view of things or that I was able to clarify facts like dates, which the teacher had got wrong. I think that is because I was not so aggressive any more.

Gradually I became more aware of my own actions and how they influence others. My temper has calmed down considerably and I also get on better with my family. The exercise taught me to be more compassionate and accepting of myself and of others.

Imagining future events in a positive way was particularly helpful.

Reflecting compassionately on myself and others and mentally rehearsing future events now helps me to deal with people I used to find hard to take. I am also better with exam situations.

Recently I went to a few job interviews and felt that they went very well. Out of four interviews I was offered three jobs. In the past I usually found the interviews rather annoying and resented the interviewers' superior behaviour. I think now that might have been because I have been putting on a rather arrogant act.

I feel more confident now because I am able to rehearse the situations mentally and therefore can act more naturally in potentially stressful situations. I believe I have changed and more people seem to like me. In the past, although having good friends, I had problems with older people in authority.

I have now taken a year out after my A-levels to do some travelling and possibly some teaching in developing countries. It is rather ironic that I am even thinking about that.

Somehow I have learned a lot about myself through the exercises and am more interested in other people. This makes me more understanding and patient.

I am planning to start uni after my year out.

Tom R., 18 years

Mental Rehearsing

> Imagination is the beginning of creation. You imagine
> what you desire; you will what you imagine; and at
> last you create what you will.
>
> *George Bernard Shaw (1856–1950)*

Mental Rehearsing is a self-guided imagination technique that allows you to picture how to manage a forthcoming event while maintaining inner security, appreciation and confidence. As you do so, you prepare the successful outcome of a situation. This will enhance your performance greatly and free you from inner doubts, fears and insecurities.

Sensualizing the event and attaching feelings of calmness, confidence and enthusiasm to it during Mental Rehearsing prepares us to experience these rehearsed feelings at the time of the actual event. We prepare ourselves to be calmer, more confident, more lovingly involved and open-minded, when the actual event arises.

This is a very powerful and highly effective technique to prepare and deal with difficult conversations, encounters and situations.

Elements of the Mental Rehearsing technique have already been introduced as part of the Heart Breathing exercise.

Enter into a state of focused relaxation

~ Choose a quiet place and time, and sit in a comfortable
position. Enter into a state of focused relaxation
with a short Heart Breathing exercise, practising the
affirmation and feelings of calmness and security.

~ As you go into a state of focused relaxation, your subconscious mind is open to learning new ways of dealing with the challenge.

Sensualize the activity from outside your body

~ Sensualize the event by looking at it from the observer perspective, as if from outside your body ('dissociation').

~ Stay calm and emotionally uninvolved.

~ Maintain Balanced Breathing throughout the whole exercise.

~ Picturing yourself from outside your body and maintaining Balanced Breathing ensures that you neutralize negative feelings and are not overwhelmed by feelings of fear and insecurity, when picturing the event.

Sensualize the activity from within your body

~ Imagine slipping inside your body and experiencing the event through your own eyes ('association').

~ Imagine the situation in as much detail as possible in order to form a complete picture. Involve as many senses as possible, such as sight, sound, smell, touch.

~ Make the images as lively, moving, bright, sharp and loud (unless it is a scene of calmness and serenity) as possible.

~ Imagine managing the situation with confidence, ease, strength, caring and calmness.

~ Imagine enjoying this activity and being pleased with
  yourself for managing it so well.

Picturing the situation as lively, bright and colourful; experiencing yourself as acting from within your body; focusing on the
feelings and emotions that are created as you imagine yourself;
being involved in the activity; all these are aspects that enhance
the effect of Mental Rehearsing on the unconscious mind.

Sensualizing the activity from within your body will enhance
your performance greatly. You will act with calmness, appreciation and confidence and learn new ways of performing during
this and any similar situation.

Sensualize the outcome and enjoy it

~ Picture how people appreciate you and your actions,
  for example with thanks or congratulations, and feel
  the joy of having succeeded.

~ Picture and experience this future as if it is happening
  right now.

~ It is important not only to visualize (sensualize)
  the positive outcome of your endeavour and its
  consequences, but also the whole process of
  rehearsing, as that will enhance performance and help
  with skill building.

On another occasion you can do the following

Using affirmations alongside your Mental Rehearsing can
enhance the development of new skills even further.

~ Contemplate a quality or skill you wish to acquire.

~ Create a strong feeling of enthusiasm or passion for this quality or skill.

~ Picture yourself managing a future situation having acquired and practised the desired quality or skill.

~ Picture the situation in as much detail as possible.

~ Try to feel a sense of achievement, enthusiasm, empowerment and joy.

~ It is important that you only choose situations that do not cause harm to yourself and others, but enhance your own and other people's wellbeing.

~ Summarize the desired outcome or skill to be achieved in simple, positive sentences and in the present tense.

~ While inhaling, hear the sentences inwardly.

~ While exhaling, speak them inwardly.

~ Repeat these sentences again and again, reducing the volume each time, then increase the volume again. (Changing the volume and focusing on the sound of the words rather than the content alone will prevent repetition becoming mechanical and therefore make the affirmation more effective.)

~ Attach the strongest possible feelings and intentions to your sensualization and affirmation to make it more alive and meaningful. This will enhance the effectiveness of the exercises considerably.

Case Study: Driving Lesson

~

Eleven years ago I had stopped driving, a few months after we moved from Germany to England.

In the fourteen years since I had my driving license I had never been a keen driver and had always been apprehensive about driving in cities. During and after my pregnancies this became even worse. I think my fears were aggravated by a very bad accident, which happened very close to our home, resulting in two deaths and severe injuries of friends and colleagues.

Now in England, I was not only confronted with city traffic and roundabouts but also left-hand driving, and, typical for this city, lots of very narrow streets. To manage traffic here one needs quite assertive driving skills, which I clearly did not have. I became more and more scared, especially of putting other people, including my children, at risk through my bad driving. Even just getting to the high street in the suburb had me breaking out in cold sweat and made my heart race. I spent ages going round and round at the roundabouts because I was too scared to change lanes. It would have been quite funny if it wasn't so sad. Finally I gave up.

Last year I started supporting my children in learning to drive. Ironically I was the one to sit next to my son, practising in his little old car just driving around the block. For the first time since I had given up driving, I thought that it would be so nice, and very useful, to drive again. Over the next weeks driving became a more accessible skill, because I saw both my children improving so fast and I became aware of their confidence in their own ability to learn what they wanted to do.

Encouraged and instructed by my husband I started to learn the Quick Coherence exercise, a technique of heart-focused breathing devised by Doc Childre ('The HeartMath Solution').

Having practised it for several weeks I moved on to the HeartSpheres exercises. I imagined and mentally rehearsed all sorts of situations and journeys. I allowed my fears to come out and live through them, in order to transform them and replace them with positive feelings of inner calmness and appreciation.

I imagined myself mastering roundabouts and traffic in general, always breathing slowly and maintaining calmness and appreciation. I became quite good at facing negative emotions with inner detachment and tranquillity.

I am now able to review difficult past events with inner calmness and detachment, and to mentally picture difficult future situations with calm confidence and appreciation.

Last autumn my husband was so convinced that I could drive again that he bought a car for our daughter and me. He bravely went with me on my first drive around the block, which must have been quite scary. Then I tried driving on my own and practised every day. In the first few weeks I did some slow breathing when getting in the car or just reminded myself of the positive feeling during my exercises. Even after smashing a wing mirror of another car in the first week of my new driving career I was still not discouraged, and I realized that my fears were gone.

For the first time in my driving life I actually enjoyed it. After about two months I also started driving my husband's sports car and really enjoyed it.

Meanwhile, whenever I come to the roundabout close by which scared me so much, it seems as if that bad experience happened to another person; it feels so unreal. The panic and fear are now completely gone.

C.G. aged 45, art student

Intuitive Conversation

> The most important thing in communication is hearing
> what isn't being said.
>
> *Anonymous*

Intuitive Conversation (or 'developing an open mind') is a process of listening and speaking which focuses on the non-verbal elements of communication and the deeper feelings, intentions and needs of the other person.

This exercise can be done during any conversation. It deepens our (social) perception and intuitive understanding of the world and allows us to live strongly in the 'here and now.' Focused attention on the 'here and now,' on our surroundings and our inner responses allows us to develop a presence of mind that applies the heart's intuitive intelligence to living in tune with our social surroundings and solving daily situations.

Enter into a state of focused relaxation

~ Choose a quiet place and time, and sit in a comfortable position.

~ Create a moment of quiet, deepening your breathing, focusing on your heart and activating feelings of calm, confidence and appreciation for the person you are listening to.

Practise listening and focus on feelings, needs and intentions

~ Empty yourself of all personal thoughts and feelings, and focus not just on the words, but also on the other person's voice, pitch, rhythm of speech, breathing, expression and gestures. Avoid any instant judgement or reflection. Take a deep interest in all the details you notice.

~ Perceive the other person's deeper feelings, needs and intentions while listening. As you focus on the feelings, needs and intentions and non-verbal expressions, you will gain intuitive understanding and insights into the other person and deepen your relationship with him/her considerably. With a little practice you will be able to recollect the content entirely, even though you have avoided focusing on it.

~ Avoid any immediate judgement or immediate emotional response. Instead give the person your undivided attention and deep interest.

Reverberation

~ Let your impressions resonate within you, paying close attention to any thoughts, feelings and images that arise within you as an inner response. You can do this during or even minutes to hours after the conversation.

Responding

> ~ When responding in conversation, maintain a mode
> of listening towards the other person, and yourself,
> and keep focus on your heart. (For more information
> about learning to talk from your heart see The Talking
> Heart, p.132.)

This exercise offers a means to go beyond our narrow self-focused experience, and enter fully into the perception and intuitive acknowledgement of another person, which leads us into a deeper conversation. Developing feelings of calmness, appreciation and inner strength in our daily encounters with other people can prepare us for emptying ourselves of all personal thoughts and feelings.

During this time we can develop a deep interest in voice, expression and gestures. Listening beyond content and concepts, we are able to focus on the other person's feelings, needs and intentions. In so doing, we refrain from critical judgements and are able to open ourselves entirely to one another. We allow our impressions to resonate within us, creating thoughts, feelings and images as an inner response. The insights achieved through this mode of perception are deeper, more intuitive and more in tune with the other person and ourselves. Listening and speaking from the heart establishes a strong rapport with the other person.

Activating positive feelings

> Happiness cannot come from without. It must come
> from within. It is not what we see and touch or that
> which others do for us which makes us happy; it is
> that which we think and feel and do, first for the other
> fellow and then for ourselves.
>
> *Helen Adams (1880–1968)*

The feelings of calmness, appreciation and inner strength developed in the HeartSpheres exercises can be activated at any time during the day, especially during and after challenging situations. You can activate certain feelings by practising Balanced Breathing whilst imagining how you inhale and exhale those feelings.

~ Focus briefly on your breathing, making it more rhythmical (see Balanced Breathing).

~ Imagine how calmness, security, appreciation, caring, inner strength or confidence is breathed into your body and mind with every inhalation, and how you share these feelings with your surrounding as you exhale.

~ Use the affirmations of the Heart Breathing exercise to intensify the feelings if so required. This can be achieved in just a few breathing cycles and will be very effective.

The activation of calmness, security, appreciation, caring, inner strength or confidence in everyday situations will help you to eliminate feelings of negativity, and allow you to refocus on the 'here and now' experience. It can directly prevent you from succumbing to negatively-loaded memories or projecting images of failure into the future. As you activate those feelings, you will not only reduce stress, but also create the physiological and psychological foundation for your intuitive heart intelligence. This allows you to develop sound judgement and creative decision-making.

Transforming disturbing emotions

Caution: Should you suffer from the effects of severe trauma then do not attempt to work on highly traumatic events without the help of a qualified therapist, as you may put yourself at risk of re-traumatization and aggravation of your symptoms.

> To exist is to change, to change is to mature, to mature is to go on creating oneself endlessly.
>
> *Henri-Louis Bergson (1859–1941)*

Disturbing emotions can have a long-term impact on physical and emotional health. As we absorb those disturbing emotions through acceptance and compassion, we have the ability to transform their energy into a positive and life-enhancing experience.

This exercise can be very helpful in improving and transforming difficult human relationships. After having been exposed to situations that bring up strong, disturbing emotions, the following steps can clear and transform the impact of those events:

Step 1: Re-experience and neutralize the negative impact of the stressful event

Choose a quiet place and time, and sit in a comfortable position. Enter into a state of focused relaxation with a short Heart Breathing exercise, practising the affirmation and feelings of calmness and security. As you go into a state of focused relaxation, your subconscious mind is open to learning new ways of dealing with the challenge. Should the rhythm of your breathing become disturbed by intense emotions, pause in your inner activity, refocus on bringing your breathing rhythm to a balance and then resume the original activity. Controlled, regular breathing allows you to stay in control of the process and avoid re-traumatizing or becoming overwhelmed by triggered emotions.

~ Recollect (visualize/sensualize) the event.
— Should the emotions, related to the event, become too strong and intense, picture yourself from outside your body, removed from the event.
— Should the emotions be weak, picture yourself as within your body and make the image animated, bright and colourful.
— You may have to work on the same event a few times, before succeeding in experiencing the emotions attached as moderately strong.
— Some people experience very strong emotions or feelings attached to the event. Other people's emotions and feelings may be very faint as they recollect the event.

~ Recognize the emotions you experience and acknowledge their nature. Identify the unmet needs which underlie those emotions.

~ Ease or intensify the emotions which are attached to the event. They should be clearly experienced but should not be overwhelming.

Step 2: Transform your emotions and change your inner attitude towards yourself and others

Create feelings of compassion for yourself (and others) while maintaining Balanced Breathing. Should you find it difficult to develop genuine feelings of compassion for yourself, then imagine the part that has led you to your negative emotional response or reaction as a hurt inner child. This hurt inner child is the underdeveloped part of your personality; we all carry it within us. Picture this hurt child within you and give it your caring and compassion in order to allow it to heal, grow and mature.

~ *Absorb* and *dissolve* the uneasy feelings in the compassion of your heart

~ *Accept* your problems and your current stage of development that will develop further.

~ *Forgive* yourself for not living up to your expectations.

Step 3: Open your heart to your intuitive intelligence

~ Empower yourself by creating an *open mind* with deep interest in what has initially been a difficult situation for you. Having calmed and eased your disturbing emotions and having developed a sense of compassion, acceptance or forgiveness, you are now ready to learn from the situation and to open yourself to your heart's intuitive intelligence.

~ To support this activity, conjure up the *feeling of inner strength* and open-mindedness while continuing Balanced Breathing.

~ Now empty your mind and *ask your heart* what the most appropriate response is to this situation.

~ *Mentally rehearse* your response in order to deal with similar situations differently in future.

The first step allows you to re-experience and then neutralize the negative impact of the stressful event.

The second step helps you to transform your emotions and change your inner attitude towards yourself and others.

The third step opens your heart to your intuitive intelligence and gives you new, creative and practical insights and social skills, which help you to act out of consideration and in a caring manner.

2. Supplementary Exercises

Developing mastery of thought

> You can't solve a problem with the same kind of thinking that created it.
>
> *Albert Einstein (1879–1955)*

The following exercises can help you to control your thoughts. Please practise these exercises when you get distracted by invading thoughts, memories and images or if you find it difficult to maintain focus and concentration. The first two exercises use imagination to enhance focus and concentration, the third exercise helps to develop consistency of clear thinking.

As you may get distracted whilst doing your HeartSpheres exercises through the flow of your thoughts or images, look at them with interest and then send them away. Redirect your attention towards your slow breathing and on your heart, before returning to the content of your exercise. Don't try to suppress your thoughts. If necessary, let them happen as you continue with your exercise. The benefit of the HeartSpheres exercises is only marginally affected by those thoughts and images.

The blue sky

This imagination can be very effective in calming your thinking and clearing your head of thoughts. Visualize thoughts as grey clouds in a blue sky. See this clearly. Gently begin to blow the clouds away with your breath. Continue blowing the clouds away until the sky is completely blue and clear.

Caduceus

The Caduceus, as a meditation symbol, was introduced by Rudolf Steiner for the above-mentioned purpose.

Two snakes entwine the staff of Hermes, the Olympian god of boundaries and of the travelers who cross the threshold. On Hermes' caduceus, the snakes are not merely duplicated for symmetry, they are paired opposites.

Concentrating on the symbol of the Caduceus is a very effective way of silencing thoughts, images and memories related to the day's events during meditation and helps you to stay focused and awake. It is most effective when practised at the beginning and end of any meditation.

Imagine a bright yellow rod entwined by a black and a white snake. The two snakes entwined on the rod cross each other at their tails and in the middle of the rod itself. Their heads meet at the top of the rod. The caduceus symbolizes the balance and the union of the sun and moon qualities within us. These qualities are representatives of male and female, day and night, wakefulness and sleep, focus and relaxation etc.

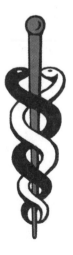

Thought control exercise

This exercise, introduced by Rudolf Steiner, helps you to develop clear and consistent thinking, which can even be maintained in situations of stress and exposure to strong emotions. It will help you to maintain calmness and allow you to deepen your capacity for clear logical thinking. Choose a simple object for your Contemplation, such as a pen, match, pencil etc. It is important to choose an object that is simple so that you have to create interest and attention through your own efforts, without being carried away. Close your eyes and start thinking about this object. Describe to yourself its material, colour and structure. Describe the way it has been made. Describe how it can be used etc. It is important to maintain focus on the object and to keep it in your mind throughout the whole exercise, so that it will be as sharply present in your mind at the end of the exercise as it was at the beginning. You can slowly extend this exercise until it lasts for approximately five minutes. Practise this exercise for five minutes every day for a period of four weeks to enhance logical thinking.

Extending sensory perception

> People only see what they are prepared to see.
>
> *Ralph Waldo Emerson (1803–82)*

> We don't see things as they are. We see them as we are.
>
> *Anaïs Nin (1903–77)*

This exercise is similar to the Intuitive Conversation, p.81. The exercise can be applied to the observation of any natural objects, and deepens our perception and intuitive understanding of nature. It also helps us to live strongly in the here and now. As we focus and direct our undivided attention towards the subject of observation, our heart's intuitive intelligence helps us to gain deep insight into the spirit of nature. The exercise outlined here is inspired by Goethe's approach to science (see Part 3. Also Ernst Lehrs, *Man and Matter,* see Bibliography).

Activation of feelings of calmness, appreciation and open-mindedness

Enter into a state of inner calmness, appreciation and open-mindedness by focusing very briefly on your breathing (see Heart Breathing exercise). This is to tune yourself into the following exercise.

Pure observation

~ *Empty* yourself of all personal thoughts and feelings.

~ *Focus* entirely on the natural object, absorbing its whole being (for example, plant, animal, sky, ocean) and engaging all your senses (sight, sound, smell, taste, warmth, touch, movement, balance.).

~ *Avoid* any judgement or reflection.

~ Take a deep *interest* in all the details whilst observing.

~ At this stage, focus on sensory perception rather than on the thoughts or inner images which arise within you.

~ By delaying judgement and interpretation of the content of your perception at this stage, you can be more open to gaining intuitive understanding and insights into what you observe, thus deepening your relationship with it considerably.

'After image'

Let your impressions resonate within you, now paying attention to any thoughts, feelings and images rising as inner response. You can do this during or even minutes to hours after the observation.

In order to support the observation process, maintain Balanced Breathing and focused relaxation during this exercise. This exercise offers a means to go beyond our narrower, self-focused experience. You will enter fully into the perception and intuitive acknowledgement of a natural object, thus leading to an extension of perception and an intuitive deepening of our understanding.

Refraining from critical (or self-critical) judgement, we can open ourselves entirely to the object of observation. This allows perceived impressions to resonate within us, creating thoughts, feelings and images which rise within us as an inner response. The insights achieved through this mode of perception will be deeper, more intuitive and therefore more in tune with the natural object and with ourselves.

Extending our perception to develop intuitive understanding of the spirit of nature considerably reduces stress, enhances our health and our vitality, creates a deep sense of joy and helps us to overcome feelings of isolation or loneliness.

3. Integrating the Exercises into Your Daily Life

Idea and experience will never coincide in the centre;
only through art and action are they united.

Johann Wolfgang von Goethe (1749–1832)

There are many ways to introduce the HeartSpheres tools into your life. The following is intended as a guide to help integrate the exercises into daily reality. Any of these elements can be adapted to your specific requirements.

Some advice

Choose a time of the day when you can be undisturbed. Avoid midday or midnight and don't practise the exercises for at least $1\,^1/_2$ hours after a main meal. The early morning after waking and/or the evening before going to sleep can be very favourable times.

Initially introduce Balanced Breathing and the affirmation of calmness and security during the first week.

Add the affirmations of caring and appreciation, strength and confidence, and balance and harmony; each of these steps can be added every one or two weeks.

Contemplation and Mental Rehearsing can be added any time you feel ready for them.

Initially you may take between fifteen to thirty minutes to perform this exercise, but don't exceed thirty minutes once or twice daily.

With increasing experience you may take only three-quarters or half the time to do this exercise satisfactorily and you can use the spare time to introduce the Inner Dialogue. Alternatively you can do the Inner Dialogue at a different time of day.

As you gain experience of these exercises, you will find the inner confidence to adapt them to your individual needs.

You can add the Reframing Past Experiences or Transforming Disturbing Emotions, whenever you want to process past traumatic experiences in order to reduce and neutralize their impact on your life.

Add the Mental Rehearsing exercise whenever you want to develop new skills or personality traits.

Listening with the Heart and Activating Positive Feelings can be practised at any time.

Important: Don't force anything and don't create expectations you may be unable to fulfil. Let the exercises develop slowly. Should you encounter difficulties with the exercise, don't be too self-critical. It is your inner attitude and your regular effort that make these exercises so powerful and effective and not how well you perform them in a particular situation. The latter will improve with time. Develop joy rather than a mere sense of duty, and avoid feelings of guilt if you don't always manage to do your exercises. Instead, just decide to try again tomorrow.

Case Study: A New Sense of Awareness

⁓

This is a brief description of the way in which I use the HeartSpheres exercises to help me manage debilitating chronic fatigue:

I started practising HeartSpheres exercises about a year ago to see if it would help me manage a problem which I have with debilitating chronic fatigue following treatment for cancer three years ago.

I was already taking complementary remedies prescribed by Dr Gruenewald to alleviate this fatigue, and wanted to explore the possibilities offered by the HeartSpheres exercises of being able to direct and harness positive thoughts and translate these into energy and healing.

After receiving 'one-to-one' tuition I started by practising an exercise called Reviewing Past Experiences. For several months I used this form of active meditation every evening and found that it helped me to achieve a very relaxed but focused frame of mind in which to review my daily activities.

I began by reviewing the day's main events including the people I had met, discussions that had taken place and any problems or difficulties which I had encountered. I was surprised to find that I could visualize and recall events in great detail whilst still maintaining a feeling of detachment and inner calm. At the close of the review I sustained this feeling of peace and calm for about five minutes whilst repeating a mantra promoting healing and affirming my personal wellbeing.

One immediate benefit was the ease with which I was able to get off to sleep at night and the quality of the sleep which I enjoyed. By finishing each day with a sense of positive achievement I had effectively drawn a line under the day's events and was able to look forward to the next day with renewed energy.

I still practise this exercise about three times a week and have found that repeated use of it brings longer term benefit, which comes from the inner objectivity which I have developed about myself and others. Learning to recognize the feelings and emotions which drain me physically or emotionally and those which energize me, helps me to plan and manage my day more constructively. It is not possible to eliminate stressful, difficult or challenging situations from life, but what I have found is that this inner sense of awareness helps me to respond to these situations more effectively. By generating a more positive personal response in a difficult or stressful situation, I am able to conserve precious energy levels and manage my day more effectively.

About nine months ago I was also introduced to the other HeartSpheres exercises and find that the

Heart Breathing exercise is a very powerful and beneficial prelude to meditation. My personal preference is to combine the affirmation of caring and appreciation with the affirmation of strength and confidence in the morning. This energizes me and helps me to build upon the benefits of a relaxed peaceful night's sleep. In the evening I prefer to combine the affirmation of calmness and peace with the affirmation of balance and harmony. I alternate this latter combination with the Reviewing Past Experiences exercise for optimum benefit.

D.W., 55 years, Human Resources Manager (recently retired)

Part 2

The Background

4. The Intelligent Heart

How to live life as a work of art, rather than as a
chaotic response to external events ...

Mihaly Csikszentmihalyi

Physiologically, the human heart maintains circulation throughout the body, helping to transport inhaled oxygen to the cells of
all organs (arterial circulation), as well as transporting toxins
and carbon dioxide away from the cells (venous circulation).
Some of this carbon dioxide is exhaled via the lungs. The heart
is not just a 'pump' however, but an organ which actively perceives the overall state of the whole organism and continually
adjusts and balances it. As such, it is the core of our physical
existence, serving us as an organ that not only regulates material processes but helps to create equilibrium between will,
emotions and cognition (thoughts and perceptions). Creating
a balance and harmony between cognition, emotion and will
within the heart leads to the development of intuitive heart
intelligence, which accesses deeper levels of practical wisdom,
love, self-determination and self-empowerment.

A state of emotional or mental imbalance often arises where
one particular force predominates in us in an unhealthy way:
perhaps our thoughts 'run away' with us, or our emotions overwhelm and threaten to submerge us; or we feel paralysed and
unable to act on any decision. The heart's role — often under
attack nowadays in our chaotic, arrhythmic lives — is to reflect
and aid our attempts and growing ability to harmonize thoughts,
feelings and actions in a living and dynamic interplay.

The link between heart and human consciousness has been known the world over for aeons. It is not for nothing that we talk of 'a heart of gold' or 'faint-hearted' or 'dying of a broken heart.' One way to observe this connection is when the heart is under attack in some way. Coronary heart disease and angina attacks are often accompanied by a deep sense of fear and anxiety, leading to fast, shallow breathing, speeded heart-rate and other symptoms. Many patients suffer moderate to severe depression for months after major heart surgery. Other organs, too, affect our consciousness and perception of ourselves and of the world, and their disorders likewise are associated with distinct changes of consciousness.

When the organism is exposed to challenging and threatening situations, it responds with a 'fight or flight response' (mediated through the sympathetic part of the autonomic nervous system). When we are in a state of acute stress, our heartbeat speeds up, our breathing becomes shallow, we may break out in a cold sweat and our skin becomes cold and pale. This physiological stress response is mediated by the sympathetic part of our autonomic nervous system. This sympathetic activity goes hand in hand with a mobilizing of energy and increased levels of alertness, but often the higher functions of judgement and decision-making can be blocked and we respond more instinctively.

During times of deep relaxation, sleep, after eating, or when we are embarrassed the heartbeat slows down, breathing becomes more abdominal (diaphragmatic), the skin becomes flushed and hot, and we perspire. This is the physiological response associated with regeneration and the rebuilding of our organism. It is mediated by the parasympathetic nervous system. Parasympathetic activity can lead us to sleepy, dream like, imaginative states of mind, leaving us open to suggestion as well as profound learning in order to accesses our unconscious mind.

When the autonomic nervous system is in balance (balance between sympathetic and parasympathetic activity), we can stay focused and alert as well as relaxed and open at the same time. This allows our conscious and unconscious mind to work in perfect partnership. In this state of balance we become creative and intuitive and are able to tap into the resources of our deeper, unconscious mind. The experiences we can have during this creative and intuitive state are then accessible to our daily consciousness. Athletes or artists call this state as living 'in the zone,' a state that is closely related to the heart balancing activity. Living 'in the zone' allows us to access the intuitive wisdom of our heart. This wisdom is made available for our day-to-day activities. As we learn to access the state of our peak performance, we can achieve an enhanced synchronization and harmonization between the functions of heart, brain and the metabolic organs (solar plexus). These all contribute to development of the heart's intuitive intelligence. This state of living 'in the zone' is also known as flow state. According to Mihaly Csikszentmihalyi, psychology professor in Claremont, California, flow is the mental state of operation in which the person:

~ is completely involved, focused, concentrating; either due to innate curiosity or as the result of training;

~ experiences a sense of ecstasy, of being outside everyday reality;

~ experiences great inner clarity, knowing what needs to be done and how well it is going;

~ knows the activity is doable, that the skills are adequate, and is neither anxious nor bored;

~ experiences a sense of serenity, has no worries about self; with a feeling of transcending ego in ways not thought possible;

~ is thoroughly focused on the present, doesn't notice time passing (timeliness);

~ is intrinsically motivated; whatever produces "flow" becomes its own reward.

(See *Flow: The Classic Work on How to Achieve Happiness* by M. Csikszentmihalyi)

The HeartSpheres exercises teach us how to access these creative states of mind with more ease, whenever we need to. We learn to live our life in balance and to access intuitive heart intelligence.

Intuitive heart intelligence harmonizes instinct (gut response), judgement (heart feeling) and common sense (intellect and knowledge). It activates the knowledge we have acquired through our past experiences, recognizes the future developmental potential and makes both available in the here and now, often within the blink of an eye. Acting out of intuitive heart intelligence means acting in harmony with past experiences, and acting in openness to future possibilities. This is a highly creative state of mind which opens us up to completely new perspectives of theoretical and practical problem solving.

It is the human heart through which the human 'I,' our core self, plays a central role in managing and transforming extreme emotions. The heart has its own autonomous nervous and hormonal network, which communicates with the brain via the afferent nerves (leading form the heart to the brain) of the autonomous nervous system. Among other things it influences the *corpus amygdale,* the brain centre of our emotional memory. Ganglions, which are part of the emotional brain, show activity of the same frequency as the heart rhythm. The heart also produces hormones such as oxytocin; this activates distinct brain function and is, for example, connected with the feeling of falling in love. The heart and brain also communicate via electromagnetic activity, as well as the mechanical pulse wave.

The exercises in this book strengthen the heart in a variety of ways, both physiologically and emotionally. Health is all about balance — for instance, between attentiveness and relaxation — and these techniques help to develop attentive and focused relaxation. This state of consciousness harmonizes dynamic heart rhythms. In stress situations, in contrast, heart rhythms become irregular and haphazard.

As Doc Childre and Howard Martin have pointed out in their book *The HeartMath Solution* (see Bibliography), experimental research has shown that there are three steps to achieving effective stress relief and autonomic nervous system balance: Balanced Breathing, heart focus and the development of positive feelings. The exercises described here integrate these three well-researched steps of emotional management and stress relief. Performing the exercises once or twice daily, or several times weekly, for a period of 15–30 minutes, develops the capacity to call up the emotional responses needed for managing stressful situations, or at least for being able to sustain a neutral state characterized by inner calmness and absence of emotional judgement.

Having achieved this state of balance — which is both emotional and physiological — we can then contemplate how to best manage the difficult situation we are in. Like a lighthouse in a stormy sea, we can learn to access the steady response of this intuitive, emotional intelligence even when battered by life's challenges.

Systematically applying the HeartSpheres exercises to our daily life can fundamentally improve challenges in our social relationships, and help to deepen our social and professional skills.

Transforming extreme emotions

The HeartSpheres exercises help to transform:

~ Stress
~ Anxiety
~ Sadness
~ Anger
~ Hyperactivity
~ Fatigue

They likewise enhance:

~ Professional performance
~ Creativity
~ Personal development
~ Intuitive insight
~ Empathy
~ Empowerment
~ Personal relationships

5. Understanding Stress

The truth is that our finest moments are most likely
to occur when we are feeling deeply uncomfortable,
unhappy, or unfulfilled. For it is only in such moments,
propelled by our discomfort, that we are likely to step
out of our ruts and start searching for different ways or
truer answers.

M. Scott-Peck

The purpose of stress

Extreme emotions such as anxiety, fear, anger and sadness have
important functions in protecting our personality and integrity
from adverse conditions. For example, the 'fight or flight' reaction when we are under threat, a function of the sympathetic
part of the autonomic nervous system. Experiencing extreme
emotions over long periods has a negative effect on our health
— especially on the autonomous nervous system, heart and
circulation and the endocrine and immune systems. Long-term
effects are cumulative and can lead to faster ageing, chronic
diseases (for example hypertension, stroke and coronary heart
disease), as well as recurrent infections or even cancer.

When stress becomes a chronic condition, as it does in many
of us in this day and age, exaggerated responses occur despite
them being inappropriate for the actual stimulus or danger.
These emotional responses are associated with deep-seated
physiological patterns that manifest strongly in breathing and
circulation. Here are some examples:

~ *Anger or embarrassment* deepen the breathing involuntarily, and push the blood to the surface of our skin (blushing). We can feel hot and restless.

~ *Anxiety or fear* make the breathing shallower and push the blood inwards (paling). This creates a feeling of cold and rigidity.

~ *Feelings of calmness and appreciation,* in contrast, deepen the breathing, making it slower and more regular. They balance the circulation, heart rhythm and nervous systems. Instead of swinging violently between the extremes of cold panic and hot fury we can start to dwell increasingly in a warm realm of heartfelt feeling and response to the world.

The use of breathing technique, sensualization and affirmation allows us to develop skills and personality traits which when faced with challenging life situations we are able to draw on. These skills allow us to utilize the positive, performance enhancing qualities of stress, and neutralize and transform health undermining and performance inhibiting effects.

Past traumatic experiences

Stressful situations are often triggered by traumatic events we have experienced in the past. These tend to be re-lived over and over again. Some traumatic experiences go back to very early childhood and usually involve a social relationship which went wrong. Basic human needs, such as intimacy, protection and caring, may have been hurt or neglected. Such traumatic experiences can cause poor self-esteem, lack of trust, lack of caring for oneself and others, raised levels of anxiety, chronic irritability and chronic unhappiness.

The HeartSpheres techniques transform traumatic experiences through reliving them consciously, and through transforming the negative emotions which are attached to them. In this process we can experience equanimity, compassion, forgiveness, and raised levels of self-esteem. New positive feelings can then be attached to the past traumatic situation through exercises which work on calm detachment, recollecting events with more tranquillity, developing understanding through appreciative thinking, feeling and compassion. By this means we are able to forgive ourselves and others, thereby releasing us from the emotional bondage. We can equally learn different patterns of inner responses to a situation, rather than continuing to expect and therefore invoke similar traumatic events. By detaching ourselves from past pain we become more available for the rich opportunities of living here and now. This process is a form of relearning and reprocessing that changes the framework in which our past influences our present and our future. The relearning and reprocessing is accompanied by a profound change within the architecture of the neuronal network of our brain. As we reprocess experiences in our mind and mentally rehearse new behaviour patterns, we are able to draw in our day-to-day experiences. Reframing Past Experiences, Inner Dialogue and Mental Rehearsing are tools for the reprocessing of past traumatic experiences.

6. Finding Clarity

As human beings, our greatness lies not so much in
being able to remake the world — that is the myth
of the atomic age — as in being able to remake
ourselves.

Mohandas Karamchand Gandhi (1869–1948)

As we have seen, negative experiences from early childhood
predispose us to extreme emotions and their negative physiological effects. These experiences can be aggravated by inher-
ited characteristics. There are a huge number of things that can
trigger extreme emotions, and these depend on our personality.
Different people respond differently in different situations. Our
reactive emotional patterns, reinforced through many years of
repetition, tend to determine our behaviour.

Our emotional responses are both learned and conditioned.
We can even become addicted to the nature of our emotional
responses, a condition known as 'stress addiction.' In his
book *Management and the Brain: An Integrative Approach to
Organizational Behaviour,* Dr Suojanen, an economist, psychologist and researcher of corporation practices, describes
the addiction to stress experienced among administrators in
both industry and government. Dr Suojanen suggests that
some managers are actually hooked on stress. They get a
'high' out of controlling people and making complex deci-
sions.

Psychology of transformation

The starting point for any inner transformation is observer consciousness. It is the process of stepping out of ourselves and observing our own thoughts, emotions, intentions and actions. We also need to be conscious of how the environment — including people close to us — reacts to our actions. Compassionate self-knowledge is the trigger for any change.

Acknowledging our weaknesses and strengths with sincerity allows us to check our core values against the reality of our daily existence. We can only embark on this process by developing active but calm detachment, appreciation (for ourselves and others) and open-mindedness about our future potential for development. The gap between our ideals and reality has to be experienced before it can be overcome. Doubt, hatred and fear are obstacles on this path. The following three steps are very helpful in bridging the gap between our ideals and the realities of life, and integrating them into our actual lives.

Step 1: Imagining and affirming ideal skills
        as specifically as possible

By contemplating the new skills we wish to develop, and imagining ourselves performing them with confidence, we can attach strong, positive feelings to such skills or desired outcomes (see Mental Rehearsing, p.75). Mental Rehearsing helps to implant the new personality trait into our will.

Step 2: Acquiring clearer knowledge of our
        environment in order to apply the skill
        in an appropriate way

A new skill is a seed of potential, but it needs planting in the right soil to flourish. We therefore have to discover the true nature of our surroundings, including the people around us, to be able to make best use of a new capacity.

Step 3: Mastering skills through repeated practice

To achieve mastery and harmony in the way we engage with our surroundings, repeated practice is needed. We need to learn how to create certain feelings or emotions in response to situations, as well as how to attach them to past, present and future experiences. This may strike some as artificial, but it is vital to be fully conscious of how we are responding, to begin with, so as to change old, negative patterns. Later these new habits will settle in us, and become a more natural response. Practice has a vital role to play here. It is like learning to ride a bicycle. Once learned you can't forget it!

7. Three Basic Skills

The point of balance is the heart. It's the foundation on which to build. Activating heart frequencies by loving and caring will balance your system, bringing in peace in the moment. It's the best antidote for restoring balance and alleviating stress.

Doc Childre

Developing a balance between calmness, appreciation and strength

To stimulate healing and transformation within ourselves and others, three basic skills are required: calmness (and security), appreciation (and caring), and inner strength and confidence are three basic skills that help to balance the activities of our consciousness: cognition, feeling and will.[*] They enhance performance through living in 'the zone' or in a 'flow state' and improve judgement and decision-making through intuitive heart intelligence. The emotional balance achieved by practising these skills are reflected in improved emotional and physical health. The HeartSpheres exercises are based on these three basic skills (core values that are applied regularly in daily life, become core skills):

---

[*] These core qualities are inspired by the work of Rudolf Steiner, an Austrian educationalist, philosopher, doctor and scientist, and founder of anthroposophy. See Rudolf Steiner, *How to Know Higher Worlds: A Modern Path of Initiation.*

Calmness and security

Developing of inner calmness, security and composure helps us to distance ourselves from traumatic events (and their associated health impacts) allowing objectivity and a healthy degree of detachment from the stressful event/trauma. Through equanimity we learn to distance ourselves from the events of life and from our fellow human beings. Without detachment we are overwhelmed by life, we over-attach ourselves to people or objects, and there is a risk of burnout. In contrast, we find if we detach ourselves too strongly, we find ourselves isolated, and lacking in interest and enthusiasm for life.

The capacity to distance ourselves, where appropriate, is essential for our emotional and social health and well being. Inner calmness neutralizes the impact extreme emotions may have on our health, judgement and decision-making. The resulting inner clarity and calmness will help us to cope better with difficult or stressful experiences in the future.

Caring and appreciation

Developing a deep sense of appreciation and caring connects us strongly with others and with life. Through appreciation we embrace the world with warm feelings and prepare ourselves to become involved through activity. As we care for, respect and appreciate ourselves and others, we heighten the perception of our own and other people's feelings and needs and prepare ourselves for compassion and forgiveness.

A lack of caring and appreciation is characterized by negativity and extreme criticism and can lead to excessive guilt feelings, in the extreme to depression, loathing and social isolation. Over-caring and uncritical, excessive appreciation in contrast can lead to dependency, fanaticism or emotional burn out. We can see calmness and security on the one side and appreciation and caring on the other, as a functional polarity. It requires balancing in order to maintain emotional and physical health.

Exercises promoting equanimity, and thus detachment, therefore need balancing with skills of caring and appreciation. Exercises that develop caring and appreciation have a strongly energizing effect. They help transform inner isolation, anger or hatred into appreciation for our own and other people's needs. We also learn forgiveness for ourselves and others.

Strength and confidence

Inner strength and confidence build on inner calmness and appreciation. Inner strength and confidence empower our will to involve itself successfully within life. We may become victim to our fears and worries, lacking in trust that our deeds may make a difference to our life and the world. Lacking in strength and confidence makes us shy away from any active involvement. If our sense of strength and confidence is too strong we can do things that lack consideration and responsibility and which we may regret later.

Inner strength and over-confidence that lack calmness and caring tend to develop towards violence and manipulation. On the other hand we require strength and confidence in order to be able to manifest our aims and values within our physical reality, giving them weight and intensity. Calmness and security as well as caring and appreciation appear weak, powerless and ineffective, if they are not accompanied by strength and confidence. Strength and confidence are made human and civilized through calm consideration and loving caring and appreciation.

Strength and confidence penetrated by calmness and caring, enables us to feel safe enough to open ourselves towards fellow human beings free of prejudice and with open-mindedness.

Freedom of prejudice (open-mindedness) is strength, cooled by reason and warmed by appreciation turned outside in.

People and life situations will reveal themselves as we temporarily give up our own thoughts, feelings and preconceived judgements in conversations. We gain intuitive insight into other people and different situations. Open-mindedness rejuvenates the body, mind and spirit. It keeps us physically and emotionally young and adaptable, and it helps us embrace life without allowing fear or anger to alienate us.

Balancing the three basic skills

To avoid one-sidedness, these three core qualities or skills need to balance each other. When they do, we develop empathy and gain deeper insights into ourselves and the world around us. Through this balance we can improve our emotional and physical health and our social relationships. When others feel we perceive and understand them better, they will also respond more positively and feel encouraged to creatively take charge of their own life. The processes involved in developing these mutually enhancing qualities depend on a continual, dynamic alternation between detachment and connection: on the one hand greater detachment from our own turbulence and distress, and greater connection with the people and the world around us; and on the other, greater connection with our own deeply-held goals and ideals, and greater detachment from negative external influences that assail us.

The healthy rhythm we establish between connection and detachment is closely related to the heart rhythms of systole (contraction) and diastole (dilation). During systole the heart muscle contracts and the blood moves from the centre (heart) to the periphery (organs). During diastole the heart muscle relaxes, allowing part of the blood to return to the heart. As the heart contracts and the blood flows to the periphery, we open ourselves to the outside world (skin, lungs); this is a similar process to the physiological expression of hot feelings like embarrassment and fury. During diastole the blood is drained slightly from the periphery allowing the blood to return partly to the heart where its quality is perceived by the heart. This process is comparable with the direction of the movement of blood in states of fear and anxiety, where we try to close ourselves off from the surrounding in order to make ourselves strong to encounter the threatening event. We connect to the world through our heart; as we inhale the blood flows to the periphery of the lungs and opens itself to the oxygen of the outside world. As we exhale the blood flows back to the centre of our body into our heart and withdraws from the world. The heart perceives the changes within the blood and responds to these changes by changing its physiology.

The human spirit connects with the world through caring and appreciation; it then detaches itself from the world through calmness and security in order to be able to process what has been experienced and transform it into knowledge and insight. After connecting with the world we need a time of detachment and awareness, of coming 'back' to ourselves, to fully absorb and digest the experience. In the morning, on awakening, we experience attachment to life; likewise we detach ourselves at night with calmness and security before we fall asleep. If we cannot maintain a dynamic balance between attachment and detachment, we risk being handicapped in fulfilling our life's aspirations or even becoming ill.

There is a strong physiological link between our breathing process and circulation. We can affect the rhythm of our heartbeat through both feelings, and the breathing process. This physiological phenomenon of influencing the heart rhythm and action through breathing is called 'respiratory arrhythmia.' As we inhale, the heartbeat speeds up, systolic activity is enhanced, and more blood flows from the centre to the periphery. As we exhale, the heartbeat slows, diastolic activity is enhanced, and more blood flows from the periphery to the centre. Regular, slow, whole chest and abdominal breathing with an equally long duration of inhalation and exhalation balances the autonomic nervous system as well as the rhythm and the action of heart and its circulation.

As we practise the HeartSpheres exercises, we create feelings of calmness and security, caring and appreciation, as well as strength and confidence in balance and harmony. The consciousness exercises and Balanced Breathing work synergistically on mind and body simultaneously, anchoring the experience of emotional balance and 'flow' deeply within our physiology.

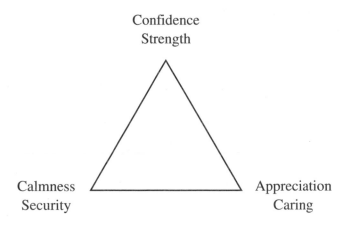

Triangle symbolizing
balance of three basic skills

8. The Techniques of Transformation

The following techniques used in this approach are presented here in overview, so that you can understand the process involved. The HeartSpheres exercises, described in Part I, are based on the following techniques:

~ Focused relaxation
~ Balanced Breathing
~ Sensualization
~ Affirmation
~ The thinking heart
~ The feeling heart
~ The talking heart

Focused relaxation

Accessing states of relaxation, while sustaining full alertness/focus and control over our inner experiences, deepens the effect of the subsequent exercises. Relaxation also helps gradually transform our personality by changing limiting beliefs, helping to create new personality traits, and social and professional skills. With repetition and practise the physiological benefits of focused relaxation become permanent and sustained. The physiological and psychological effects of focused relaxation are:

~ *Effects on the brain:* Focused relaxation changes the
   brain's activity from predominantly beta brainwaves,
   which process sensory perception, to increased
   alpha, theta and delta brainwave activity. These
   brain activity patterns are found when day-dreaming

(alpha), falling asleep (theta), upon awakening (theta), during vivid dreaming in REM sleep (theta), and during deep, dreamless and regenerating sleep (delta). These brainwaves are apparent in EEG trials, which measure the brain's electrical activity in different states of consciousness. The meditating person learns to access these states of altered consciousness at will, maintaining full alertness and control, and learns to unite day consciousness with night consciousness.

~ *Effects on the body:* The autonomic nervous system comes into balance. Stress-induced sympathetic activity will diminish, and regenerating parasympathetic activity will increase accordingly. The breathing rhythm slows down and deepens. The heartbeat slows down and becomes more rhythmical, showing increased coherence. The blood pressure is reduced. Hormone levels change: stress hormones (such as adrenaline and cortisol) reduce whilst regenerating hormones (such as DHEA) increase. The immune system enhances its protective activity. Sleep deepens and becomes more refreshing.

~ *Effects on consciousness:* The conscious and subconscious mind work closely together. In focused relaxation we can experience the higher self and its creative intentions that enter deeply into the human personality. These intentions are aided by visualization and affirmation exercises.

~ *Effects on imagery and affirmations:* Focused relaxation amplifies the power of imagery and affirmations. This helps realize our intentions.

Balanced Breathing

Breathing reflects our emotions

Breathing is a continuous, vital function that works automatically. We don't have to be aware of it, but we can control it consciously. Breathing is a physical reflection of our feelings and emotions, too. Are we stressed, anxious, happy, nervous, or exerting ourselves? Pay attention to your breathing and you will know the answer at once.

Cold emotions, such as anxiety and fear, make breathing shallow. Hot emotions, such as anger and embarrassment, make breathing involuntarily deep. During the day we breathe more shallowly than at night. During intellectual work such as studying, the breath becomes shallow and our skin becomes cold. When we are engaged in imaginative creative activities or physical activity, the breath deepens and the skin becomes warm.

In a deeply relaxed or sleeping state, we usually breathe from our diaphragm, but expand our ribcage and chest too. The diaphragm is a thin, muscular partition between the chest and abdomen. It is sensitive to tension and reacts to strong emotions, such as anxiety and fear. A cramped diaphragm results in a cramped and imperfect way of breathing. As the diaphragm contracts, it moves down, and we then breathe into our abdomen. The result is that air streams into our lungs. The deeper the diaphragm is pushed down during breathing, the more air will enter our lungs. When we exhale, the diaphragm relaxes and moves up. It is important to allow chest, ribs and the abdomen to expand as you inhale. The inhalation and exhalation should be equally long and slow, expanding your abdomen and thorax (chest) on inhalation. A breathing rhythm which is slowly reduced to approximately six cycles per minute (inhalation: 4–5 seconds / exhalation: 4–5 seconds) can help to reduce stress instantly, deepen relaxation and focus and balance your autonomic nervous system.

As Doc Childre and his team have found (see *The HeartMath Solution),* focusing on the heart while breathing can further enhance the balancing effect of slow, regular breathing. Via the breathing process, we can learn to control and transform our emotional responses. Practising slow and regular breathing and concentration on heart and body periphery combined with sensualization and/or affirmation techniques and positive feelings helps generate physical and emotional health as it balances our autonomic nervous system activity. The combination of breathing, concentration on heart and body periphery and emotional/mental exercises can create new positive physiological patterns, and our body and mind can develop and learn new skills and neurological pathways. This means we can gradually transform the benefits into deeper personality traits and skills.

Sensualization

> There is a law in psychology that if you form a picture
> in your mind of what you would like to be, and you
> keep and hold that picture there long enough, you will
> soon become exactly as you have been thinking.
>
> *William James (1842–1910)*

Sensualization (creating vivid sensory images involving as many senses as possible, such as sight, hearing, touch, taste, smell, movement etc.) is applied, disciplined imagination. What we habitually imagine is often what we come to believe, and hence what we create in our lives. Effective sensualization takes place when we are in focused relaxation. During sensualization, you relax and talk to or direct your inner self to create a chosen image within your mind. Sensualization and memory techniques focus the mind and engage the creative will. Research on guided imagery proves its effectiveness in managing stress-related conditions. Other studies show that focusing the imagination in specific ways can be calming, encouraging, mood-modulating, pain relieving, and may even speed up physical and emotional healing.

Images are especially effective when they are multi-sensory. Imagery involving seeing, hearing, tasting, smelling and even touching is more effective than just visualizing. For instance, as you imagine yourself in a healing sanctuary/idyllic setting you can 'feel' the wind gently blowing through your hair, 'hear' its gentle whisper, 'smell' the fragrance of flowers growing nearby and 'taste' the saltiness of the sea.

Sensualization frees our body and emotions, thus promoting healing. When we take inner journeys, we rearrange our inner landscape. We learn to accept our past, to live in our present, and to take charge of creating our future. As artists and poets know, the unconscious is a deep source of energy and creativity which we can learn to draw on, raising its treasures and hidden potency to the light of awareness. Life becomes healthier and richer if we can mediate in this way between dream and daylight reality. Imaginative activity is a form of active, deepened daydreaming. It allows us to access deep-seated memories, emotions and beliefs. It also allows us to revisit past experiences, to re-experience them in a detached and calm manner and then to re-process them by attaching new feelings and emotions to them. Daydreaming techniques allow us to mentally rehearse and acquire new inner skills.

Sensualization guidelines

Always sensualize (i.e. vividly imagine sensory qualities) as if the future were happening now. Our subconscious takes everything literally. When you visualize yourself as healthy, calm, loving and strong now, then the process of transformation will begin NOW.

Sensualize in as detailed a way as possible, and make images as vivid and realistic as you can. See colours and shapes, examine your mental image from various viewpoints and make it three-dimensional. Involve as many senses as possible — sight, sound, touch, warmth, smell. The more senses you involve, the more real the image will be for your subconscious.

Feel the emotions associated with each image — calmness, security, caring, appreciation, strength, joy, happiness, a sense of fulfilment. Sustain these feelings during the whole sensualization exercise.

Always sensualize with the purpose of improving everybody's lives, even the state of the whole world! The exercises will be more beneficial for yourself and anyone involved.

Sensualization works best when you are relaxed, as you are more open to your own suggestion and are less hindered by distracting thoughts.

Repeat the sensualization as frequently as you can.

Sensualization has a stronger effect when combined with affirmation (see Affirmation, below).

Believe that you are capable of sensualizing. Create positive affirmations like 'I can visualize' and avoid negative affirmations, like 'I can't do it.'

Problems with sensualizing and their resolution

If you have difficulties sensualizing, be patient with yourself. This capacity will develop with practice. One way in is to tell yourself what it is that you wish to see. Make this description as detailed as you can. As you do this, the image or sensory experience will come into sharper focus so that your 'image' gradually becomes more and more vivid. After a while, silence your thinking and allow the image or imaginative sensory experience to 'blossom.' Different people have different dominant senses, but the most common is the sense of sight. This is why the process of visualization works well for most people. Some, however, may have a dominant sense of touch, movement, hearing or smell. These people may have difficulty 'visualizing' but may be able to accurately imagine sounds, smells, taste, touch or movement. It is important for them to incorporate these senses into their 'mental experience.' People born blind, for example, can still engage in creative sensualization, creating an imaginative experience by drawing on their sense of smell, hearing, taste and touch.

You can exercise your weaker, non-dominant senses through regular practice and activity, deciding for instance to focus on one sense in particular that is not yet strongly developed in you.

Affirmation

> You must begin to think of yourself as becoming the person you want to be.
>
> *David Viscott (1938–96)*

Affirmations are strong, positive and feeling-rich statements. They can relate to yourself and others, or situations and experiences you wish to invoke in your life. As affirmations become rooted in our subconscious, they act as powerful regulators of our beliefs and behaviours. When we are in a deep, focused state of relaxation we can suggest behaviour-changing ideas to our subconscious mind. Used in this way, affirmations transform negative views about ourselves, our motives, values and attitudes into positive ones. By harnessing the power of the subconscious to influence our conscious mind and vice versa, we achieve a sustainable change in our attitude towards life, and in our habitual responses.

There are three essential elements to make affirmation effective:

1. *Desire:* you must truly want it.

2. *Belief:* you must believe it is possible for you.

3. *Acceptance:* you must be willing to accept that the situation will happen, and that it will benefit you and others.

Affirmations are particularly effective during or at the end of sensualization sessions. Through repetition they become increasingly effective. Sensualization and affirmation combined enable us to shape our future.

Preparing your mind for affirmation (and sensualization)

Connect with your intent:
Define what you really desire to manifest in your life — your core values (see Core Values in Part 1). For example, the initial steps of the HeartSpheres techniques use qualities such as these:

~ Inner calmness, serenity and security

~ Appreciation, caring, enthusiasm and compassion

~ Open-mindedness and freedom from premature judgement

~ Strength, empowerment, confidence and positive actions

~ Transforming my past and forgiving myself and others

~ Preparing the future and acquiring new skills

Reflect upon these qualities and then ask yourself sincerely: Will this really make me happy, and harm no one else? If you answer 'Yes!' then direct your will to give energy to your intent. Generate the strong feelings related to the affirmation and try to sustain them during the exercise, and also at other times.

The thinking heart

> All truly wise thoughts have been thought already
> thousands of times; but to make them truly ours, we
> must think them over again honestly, till they take root
> in our personal experience.
>
> *Johann Wolfgang von Goethe (1749–1832)*

Contemplating our own and other people's emotions, behaviours and unmet needs can lead to a deep sense of appreciation and compassion for ourselves and others. These feelings are generated via thinking and can help us transform our negative or shadow qualities into virtues through acceptance and forgiveness. Contemplation is often experienced like an inner conversation with our true self (see Inner Dialogue, p.51). As we contemplate our core values such as calmness, caring, compassion etc., we connect our thoughts with feelings and fire them with passion and enthusiasm and penetrate them with our intentions (see Accessing Core Values, p.45). Contemplating the content of your affirmations charges them and makes them a lot more effective (Heart Breathing exercises). Contemplation is a strongly energizing activity.

The feeling heart

> The best and most beautiful things in the world cannot be seen or even touched. They must be felt with the heart.
>
> *Helen Adams Keller (1880–1968)*

In order to transform extreme and disturbing emotions, such as anxiety, fear, anger, resentment, worry and sadness in daily life, we need to be able to name them and to admit them. After all, we are only able to change what we recognize.

Easing these emotions can be achieved through breathing and visualization techniques that go hand-in-hand with developing and sustaining feelings of calm detachment. This already helps us to neutralize the psychological and physiological effect of these emotions.

In a next step we can transform these emotions by developing a deep sense of appreciation and compassion for ourselves and others. As the power of calmness and security helps us to find distance and neutrality, the power of caring and compassion helps us to transform the emotions through forgiving ourselves and others. By attaching those two emotional responses (calmness and caring) to remembered, imagined or mentally rehearsed life events, we can create new ways of responding emotionally to the challenges of daily experiences.

Acting out of inner calmness and peacefulness as well as out of compassionate love, we need to empower our will and open up for our intuitive heart intelligence. We can rehearse our new skills mentally and enhance this experience by creating feelings of inner strength and empowerment. We can open our heart to our fellow human beings by learning to listen with our heart and our open mind.

Extreme emotions are vital for our survival. They help us to assert and protect ourselves in dangerous and adverse environments. Often we learn to invoke them in childhood to deal with threatening situations, but then they remain in us as habit when they are no longer appropriate. For example we may feel suspicious when someone makes a genuinely kind gesture towards us. It is not easy to influence such deep-seated emotional reactions since we still unconsciously believe them to be essential to our survival. The HeartSpheres exercises counter such deeply ingrained but inappropriate survival responses through relaxation techniques, breathing techniques, emotional management exercises, sensualization and affirmation, in order to create long-term changes in behaviour, emotional insight and response.

The following graph gives and overview of the relationship between core values and HeartSpheres exercises:

	Core skills (heart virtues)	Processes	HeartSpheres tools
Acknowledging disturbing feelings	Experiencing and naming our feelings	Self-knowledge	Accessing core values and identifying areas of concern
Neutralizing disturbing feelings	Inner and outer calmness, security	Detachment	Heart Breathing exercise, Inner Dialogue, Reframing Past Experiences
Transforming disturbing feelings	Appreciation, caring and compassion	Attachment	Heart Breathing exercise, Inner Dialogue
Developing new virtues and skills	Empowerment and open-mindedness	Habit building, intuition	Heart Breathing exercise, Inner Dialogue, Mental Rehearsing, Intuitive Conversation

The talking heart

> Our voices tell our life stories; they are the very blue-
> print of our psyche and therefore how we use our voice
> can utterly change our lives.
>
> *Stewart Pearce*

Stewart Pearce is an internationally renowned voice coach. He is Master of Voice at Shakespeare's Globe Theatre and Head of Voice at the Drama Centre in London. In his acclaimed book *The Alchemy of Voice,* Pearce introduces a training path of voice development that leads to the ability to talk with self-confidence, authority, caring and intuitive heartfelt insight. The straightforward but highly effective technique helps to funda-mentally change and improve both our ability for perceiving other human beings and our own capacity for self-expression.

Having worked with him, the author has come to recognize how important it is not only to develop the inner culture of the heart, but to connect the power of the heart with the way we listen and speak. The author has learned that talking from the heart truly is a spiritual path.

The author would like to share three areas of Pearce's teach-ing which have been particularly inspiring for him:

~ Listening and staying receptive to ourselves and others whilst talking.

~ Personalizing the content we talk about by connecting it with our feelings and sharing our feelings with others as we talk.

~ Staying connected with our heart while we are talking.

To work on achieving the latter the author has been practising an exercise, published in Pearce's book, that leads towards finding and working with what he calls your 'Signature Sound.' Pearce describes the heart chakra as the 'lotus of the Signature Sound.'

The Signature Sound is the sound that, when intoned, creates a resonance within our heart region. Learning to speak with a pitch of voice that oscillates close to the Signature Sound will give your voice the balance between lightness and gravity that can make it resound and reverberate for others — and in fact speak to their heart.

The author has adapted the following exercise, based on Stewart Pearce's 'Sound Centering Sequence,' to harmonize with the Heart Breathing exercise.

This exercise will help you to identify your Signature Sound and to practise and strengthen your capacity to draw on it when speaking.

~ Sit on a chair, upright, your spine aligned and your feet firmly on the ground.

~ Practise Heart Breathing as described in the preparation of the Heart Breathing exercise.

~ Imagine a beam of light radiating from your heart through your head into the universe.

~ Imagine a beam of light radiating from your heart through the base of your spine into the centre of the earth.

~ Continue with your Heart Breathing.

~ Then sound and repeat the following ...

Sound	as in	Feel the resonance in your
HAW	hawk	Pelvis
HOO	food	Solar plexus
HOW	down	Larynx (throat)
HEE	me	Forehead
HAA	calm	Heart

~ Listen to a distant sound.

~ Connect with all your senses and feel truly *present*.

Practising this sound sequence daily will allow you to strengthen your relationship with your Signature Sound.

The following tips can assist in talking with the Signature Sound:

~ Try to talk with a voice pitched around the signature note as centre.

~ Imagine that your heart transforms into a larynx to create your voice.

~ Listen inwardly as you talk whilst continuing to perceive the other person.

~ When you talk, try to focus slightly more on the vowels, as they carry the music of your voice and express your true feelings.

~ Stay connected with your heart and feel, what you speak.

Additional advice

Regularly reciting vowel-rich poetry, such as Shakespearean sonnets, can deepen your skill in speaking from your heart. In the work of inspired poets and writers, poetic speech and its sounds embody more than mere meaning. When listening to or reciting poetic speech, something deep is touched within our hearts: this can be experienced as a yearning for a connection with our higher self. What touches us so deeply is the music of poetic speech. The sound qualities — pitch, rhythm, and so on — move us and engage our feelings. The music of speech and its richness of imagery have the power to awaken our heart from its deep sleep, like the Sleeping Beauty when the prince kisses her. Awakening within our heart connects us deeply with our higher self, our spiritual entity, and the true core of our being.

In ancient cultures speech was more than a medium of mere communication. It was considered to be a micro-image of the creative power of God, the creative Word, and every natural creature was considered to have its own true and inherent name. 'Reading in the book of nature' and engaging in the creative act of naming were ways in which early peoples could tune and align themselves with the natural world. The creative power of speech was experienced as so powerful that blessings, curses or magic spells had a decisive impact on the human soul. From these ancient cultures stems the practice of using mantric meditation that focuses on the sound quality of a word. Meditating on certain sounds was felt to reconnect the human soul and spirit with the world of its origin and the forces that created us.

We have lost the power of speech over time. Nowadays speech tends to come from the head rather than from the heart and is not carried by an enlivening power of breath. Great writers like Shakespeare and Goethe maintain closeness to the origins of speech. They are magicians of the word, with the power to awaken the higher self within our hearts. That's why listening to or reciting their words seems to elevate and reconnect us.

Reciting poetry by great writers can help us to connect deeply with our heart, the home of our spiritual self, when their words are borne on the stream of our enhanced, heart-connected breathing.

Breath work, listening to poetry and reciting it are tools used to help you find your signature note, and connect your speech to your heart. When more experienced, you can use the signature note to hear or silently sound the affirmations of the Heart Breathing exercise, which ultimately will make them more effective.

Part 3

Origins and Related Approaches

9. The Roots

This is the highest wisdom that I own; freedom and life are earned by those alone who conquer them each day anew.

Johann Wolfgang von Goethe (1749–1832)

The HeartSpheres approach draws on three sources of inspiration, which are described below.

In their book *Transforming Stress: The HeartMath Solution for Relieving Worry, Fatigue, And Tension,* Doc Childre and Deborah Rozman introduce a simple and effective method for transforming stress. The HeartMath method is based on invoking positive feelings such as appreciation, caring, or compassion. In conjunction with heart-focused regulation of the breathing process, this can create a health-promoting balance within the autonomic nervous system. This balancing of the autonomic nervous system is detectable in changes of the patterns of heart rhythms (Heart Rate Variability). Associated with the balancing of the autonomic nervous system are a number of neural, hormonal and biochemical changes that reduce and transform stress, fear and anger and lead to greater wellbeing and health.

The HeartMath Institute developed a number of exercises that help to manage stress, transforming extreme emotions and develop intuitive heart intelligence. Some of these exercises, such as Quick Coherence, Freeze-Framing, Attitude Breathing, Heart-Lock-in and Cut-Thru have been applied successfully in fields as diverse as personal development, education, health and corporate business. These techniques are based on the three core activities: regulated breathing, heart focus, and activating positive feelings such as appreciation. HeartMath provides an invaluable model for a profound understanding of the physiology and psychology of stress and stress release. HeartMath introduces a psycho-physiological understanding of stress release based on the experience that autonomic nervous system balance can be achieved through regular breathing, focus on the heart, and the simultaneous creating and sustaining of positive feelings. It considers managing extreme emotions as an important pathway towards developing intuitive heart intelligence (emotional intelligence). These HeartMath techniques have been of help to many people all over the world. (See *The HeartMath Solution,* Childre and Martin, v. Bibliography)

The HeartSpheres approach is also inspired by the psychological research of Marshall Rosenberg, the founder of a method of human interaction, called Nonviolent Communication (NVC). Nonviolent Communication is based on a non-judgemental approach to our fellow human beings and on empathetic perception and communication of our own and other people's feelings and unmet needs. (See Chapter 12, p.149.)

The HeartSpheres exercises were developed through a Goethean understanding of natural science and human consciousness. (See Chapter 10, p.143.) The HeartSpheres approach is, equally, inspired by Rudolf Steiner's research on spiritual development, human physiology and psychosomatic conditions. (See below.)

While informed and inspired by all three approaches, HeartSpheres has developed a system of exercises which, despite certain overlaps, have techniques distinctive from those of Steiner, Childre and Rosenberg. The methods can complement each other, and elements of the one or the other approach may suit different people better.

Knowledge of the heart as an organ of wisdom, love and strength, and as the seat of our higher self, is based on the

ancient traditions of many cultures. The importance of culti-
vating heart forces so as to make them, once again, the core
and foundation of our human existence, was central to Rudolf
Steiner's anthroposophy or science of the spirit. In lectures held
during the early years of the twentieth century he described the
importance of developing heart intelligence. In this context he
developed a number of exercises, including the 'six accompa-
nying exercises' — which I consider very important. Rudolf
Steiner foresaw that heart intelligence and its development
would be a precondition for solving increasing social problems
facing humanity around the turn of the millennium and beyond.
Rudolf Steiner acknowledged breathing and circulation as the
physiological basis of our emotions and the heart as a central
organ mediating between breathing and circulation. In other
exercises, he proposed regulation of the breathing process during meditative activity as a means of transforming and mastering human emotions.

In cooperation with a number of doctors, Rudolf Steiner
founded a medical system — anthroposophic medicine — as
an extension to mainstream medicine. Within this system of
medicine, therapeutic interventions aim to balance and harmonize pathological imbalances in the organism via the breathing
process, which, together with the human heart and its rhythm
as a centre of balance, harmony and health, underlies all healing. Based on Steiner's research, the HeartSpheres approach
sees the human heart as a central organ of healing and balance,
through which cognition, emotions and will, and their physiological correlates, can be balanced with the help of the breathing process and certain core qualities.

These core qualities are inner calmness and security (head),
caring and appreciation (heart), strength and confidence (will).
Activating, balancing and harmonizing these in many ways
polar qualities creates an equilibrium which, physiologically,
resembles a high degree of harmony between heart rhythm,

and central and autonomic nervous systems. The HeartSpheres approach recognizes too that a further balance has to be achieved — the balance between 'I' and 'world,' or 'inner' and 'outer,' or 'me' and 'you.' We need such balance so as not to lose our own identity in contact with the world, and equally so as not to close ourselves off too much in inner solitude. This balance is developed through the above described core values and through the specific nature of the HeartSpheres exercises. With time HeartSpheres exercises deeply root these core values not only within our feeling life, but in our thinking, will and also in our actions.

10. Goethe's Scientific Research Method

Science arose from poetry... when times change the two can meet again on a higher level as friends.

Johann Wolfgang von Goethe (1749–1832)

HeartSpheres draws, less directly perhaps but nevertheless profoundly, on the ideas of the eighteenth century German thinker and writer, Johann Wolfgang von Goethe. Goethe's writings on natural science are very little known, but in his studies on light, colour, botany, meteorology and human anatomy he developed a method of research which can help open a spiritual dimension in our experience of nature and the human being. Goethe's method is less an analytical than a synthetic one. Rather than immediately judging the content of our perceptions, his approach allows the objects and phenomena of nature — such as the development of a plant or the changes of the clouds of the sky — to live within the human soul and sensibility, so that the changing images produced in us in this way develop, unfold and metamorphose in time. Experiencing within the human soul this process of waxing and waning of organic life allows the marriage of two opposite poles of human nature: active observation and exact sensorial imagination. Goethe called this new skill and research tool *Anschauende Urteilskraft,* which very loosely translated means the power of intuitive judgement drawing on creative perception. This refers, in other words, to our ability to acquire insights by experiencing the content of perception in a dynamic way.

In applying this inner activity to researching organic nature one learns to experience the development of organic life in terms of fundamental polarities such as birth and death, waxing and waning, light and darkness, straight line and curve etc.

Any metamorphosis of organic life appears to result from a struggle between opposite form tendencies — such as straight line and curve. One can, for example, see this in the polarity between sperm and ovum; or, in the plant, between upward-striving vertical tendencies (stem) and outspreading horizontal tendencies (leaf). The imaginative capacities of the human soul participate in this interplay of opposites and learn to inwardly recreate the world of natural phenomena, instead of just researching the dead products of life. This is, broadly, the difference between an understanding derived from dissection and anatomy and one which enters into the dynamic of living processes. In experiencing life as an organic development in time, nature's laws and synthesizing forces can reveal themselves in a different manner, allowing the researcher to participate inwardly in the process of creation. Applied to researching the human constitution in illness and health, this method offers insights that complement modern scientific research. The same method applied to the human mind and emotions leads us to an understanding of human soul life between the polarities of cognition (perception, concept and image formation) and activity (force, instinct, desire, drive).

This tension between the two poles of intellectual onlooker consciousness on the one hand, and active involvement in changing the world or satisfying our physical and emotional needs on the other, is mediated by our feelings and emotions.

Feelings and emotions live between sympathy, which embraces the world and stimulates activity, and antipathy, which creates an emotional distance and helps us to be awake and attentive in our cognition. (The terms sympathy and antipathy are far broader and less subjectively coloured than our common understanding of them; sympathy and antipathy can be seen as fundamental forces imbuing all activity in both conscious and unconscious ways and mediate between cognition and will.)

How to apply this method to the art of healing can be studied in Victor Bott's *Introduction to Anthroposophical Medicine — Extending the Art of Healing* (see Bibliography).

11. The HeartMan Technology

The HeartMan (Measurement of the autonomic nervous system) conducts a 24-hour ECG and uses Heart Rate Variability (HRV) as a diagnostic and prognostic tool for heart attack, diabetes and other serious illnesses. The HeartMan has been developed and researched by Professor Max Moser, a medical physiologist at the University of Graz, Austria. The medical measurements of cosmonauts, invited by the Russian space medicine group for 9 missions (Austro-Mir project), were the starting point of the HeartMan project.

The HeartMan creates an autochrone image that is the result of monitoring HRV and other rhythms throughout the day and night. This allows the objective evaluation of the degree of stress during daily activity, the quality of sleep via ECG measurements and the fitness of the person.

This test objectively evaluates the efficacy of stress management techniques, therapies, preventative-medical applications and lifestyle changes. The test results can also motivate people to change their lifestyle.

A biofeedback system (hardware, software and training programme) to enhance heart-rate variability and coherence, and to monitor the long-term effect of the exercises, as well as the state of health, is currently being developed in collaboration between Professor Max Moser (Institute for Non-invasive Diagnostic, IND), Dr. Peter Gruenewald and HeartBalance GMBH. Health professionals, psychologists, coaches and clients will be able to use this biofeedback system.

For more information on the HeartMan technology please visit *www.heartbalance.org*

12. Transforming Conflict

All violence is the result of people tricking themselves
into believing that their pain derives from other people
and that consequently those people deserve to be
punished.

Marshall Rosenberg

Peace is not the absence of conflict but the presence of
creative alternatives for responding to conflict — alternatives to passive or aggressive responses, alternatives
to violence.

Dorothy Thompson

Three modes of response

In his book, *Healing without Freud and Prozac,* David Servan-
Schreiber describes three types of behaviour that arise when we
are faced with conflict situations of any kind. All three types of
behaviour can manifest singly or in any combination:

Passive or passive-aggressive behaviour

Passive or passive-aggressive behaviour is the most common
behaviour in our society, experienced for example both in fami-
lies and in the workplace. Frequently it is shown by people who
consider themselves to be 'sensitive,' 'respectful of others,' 'not
wanting to rock the boat,' or 'preferring to give rather than to
receive.' As a result of this behaviour people are likely to feel
'used' and 'abused,' and to develop resentment.

Aggressive behaviour

'Aggressive behaviour' is typically, but by no means solely, masculine. It often leads to substantial damage of human relationships, such as divorce, dismissal from jobs or even physical violence and abuse. This behaviour can be a major cause of high blood pressure and cardio-vascular disease in the aggressive person, but can also be damaging for those around them.

Nonviolent assertive communication

This behaviour is assertive without being confrontational or aggressive. It acknowledges our own limits and remains respectful of the needs of others.

If this is not already our natural way of responding towards others, it can certainly be learned. (See Nonviolent Communication below.)

The four apocalyptic horsemen

> In the last decade or so, science has discovered a tremendous amount about the role emotions play in our lives. Researchers have found that even more than IQ, your emotional awareness and abilities to handle feelings will determine your success and happiness in all walks of life, including family relationships.
>
> *John Gottman*

In his book, *Why Marriages Succeed or Fail,* John Gottman states that there is no lasting relationship without chronic conflict. Gottman considers the absence of conflict as a sign of an emotional distance so great as to preclude an authentic relationship. (John Gottman is world renowned for his work on marital stability and divorce prediction, involving the study of emotions, physiology, and communication.)

Our emotional brain is most afflicted by feeling emotionally cut off from those we are most attached to. Once the emotional brain is aroused, it turns off the cognitive brain's ability to reason rationally. This 'emotional flooding' leads to thinking and acting only in terms of defence and attack. One no longer looks for responses to restore calmness to the situation. According to Gottman there are four apocalyptic horsemen, which are four attitudes that can be destructive in all relationships. These attitudes activate the emotional brain of the other person to such an extent that the other party can only see fighting or withdrawal as a response. Gottman found that the Four Horseman symptoms allowed his team to predict divorce with 85% accuracy.

Criticism

Criticizing someone's character instead of simply stating the grievance:

Criticism: 'You are late. You only think of yourself.'
Grievance: 'I am lonely and upset when I wait for you like this.'

If we criticize the other person rather than expressing a legitimate grievance, we may not be heard and may generate resentment and a counterattack.

Contempt

Insulting other people; sarcasm; facial expressions can be all it needs to communicate contempt (eyes rolling towards the ceiling, corners of the mouth turned down with eyes narrowing in reaction to the other person.) These signals make a peaceful solution practically impossible.

Any attack or counter-attack can only lead to two possible outcomes:

~ It can provoke an escalation of violence.

~ We may overwhelm the other person and force them to surrender. But the victory leaves the other wounded and sore, and this wound widens the emotional gap and makes living together more difficult.

Defensiveness

Becoming defensive is a general way of fighting off a perceived attack. Unfortunately, defensiveness usually includes denying responsibility for the problem, and this fuels the flames of conflict because it says the other person is the guilty party.

Stonewalling

After months of criticism, of attacks and counterattacks some people will choose 'flight' and will emotionally withdraw. While one person still seeks contact and offers talk, the other avoids communication. The one who feels ignored, tries to make himself or herself heard by shouting. Physical violence can be a desperate attempt to reconnect with the other who has left the scene, to try to make them hear what we are experiencing emotionally, to make them feel our pain. Emotional withdrawal is not an effective way to deal with conflicts. It often leads to the end of the relationship.

Nonviolent Communication

> The Indian philosopher J. Krishnamurti once remarked
> that observing without evaluating is the highest form
> of human intelligence. When I first read this statement,
> the thought, 'What nonsense!' shot through my mind
> before I realized that I had just made an evaluation.
>
> *Marshall Rosenberg*

Psychologist Marshall Rosenberg, author of Nonviolent Communication (see Bibliography), has come to the following conclusion about what to strive for in order to maintain a healthy relationship:

Judgement has to be replaced by an objective statement of facts. The more specific we are the better. The other person will then rather react to our words as a legitimate attempt to communicate than as an attack.

We need to avoid any judgement of the other, but instead focus entirely on what we feel. This reservation of judgement is the master key to emotional communication.

If I talk about what I feel, nobody can argue with me. The whole point is to describe the situation with sentences beginning with 'I' rather than 'you.' By talking about myself, and only about myself, I am no longer criticizing the other person. I am not attacking either. I am expressing my feelings, and therefore I am being authentic and open.

If I am skilled and really honest with myself, I can even go as far as to expose my vulnerability by showing how the other person has hurt me. The honesty can often disarm the adversary. The other person will want to cooperate if that person is interested in the relationship.

One should talk only about two things: what has just taken place — objectively and therefore beyond judgement — and what feelings one experienced in response.

It is even more effective not only to say what I feel, but also to express the unmet needs we have.

Nonviolent Communication (NVC) is a form of compassionate communication. It helps us to inspire compassion in others and to respond compassionately to others and to ourselves. Through its emphasis on deep listening — to ourselves as well as others — NVC fosters respect, attentiveness and empathy, and engenders a mutual desire to give from the heart.

Forgiveness therapy

We know from personal experience that dealing with relationship stress can have a major negative impact on our emotional wellbeing and physical health.

It is well known that recovery from relationship stress is slower than from any other stress. Susceptibility to certain triggers of interpersonal stress can be long-lasting.

A worst-case scenario presents itself wherein both parties believe that the other has behaved wrongly, and they themselves have not contributed to the problem. This often causes a gridlock situation. It is particularly problematic if the individual is a part of day-to-day life (spouse, child, co-worker), as we are continually reminded of the unresolved conflict or past wrongdoing. Long-term stress will take its toll on our emotional and physiological health, even though we believe that we are right or that our anger is justified.

The situation can change for the better, if one party decides that maintaining the relationship is more important than being right or wrong or that the other person is guilty. Taking the perspective of the other person is a major defining characteristic of a lasting marriage.

People, who have been in traumatizing, abusive or emotionally draining relationships, very often suffer with long-term emotional distress. Lack of emotional resolution by the victim is considered a contributory factor in extensive health problems, independent of the degree of empathy the person may receive. One way out is to resolve the conflict, and reduce or transform understandable anger, frustration, upset and fear through forgiveness.

If we apply forgiveness as a conflict resolution tool, we maintain control over the process, as the other party need not be involved at all.

Through forgiving, we learn to let go of and to transform negative thoughts, feelings and behaviours. At the same time we develop more compassionate understanding for the offending party.

Research published by Chapman (2001)[*] applied a forgiveness learning programme to seventeen male forensic patients who had been abused, and found that, as a result of this programme, forgiveness, hope and self-esteem were significantly increased in this patient group.

The treatment programme included four distinct phases:

~ *Uncovering phase:* dealing with feelings of hurt,
    working through shame, anger etc.

[*] See Linden 2005, pp.101–2.

~ *Commitment phase:* realizing that past strategies have failed, considering forgiveness as an option.

~ *Work phase:* attempting to see the wrong doer with new eyes, developing empathy.

~ *Deepening phase:* finding meaning in surrendering by accepting the past event, realization of not being alone, putting into perspective, taking significance out, shifting away negative feelings to greater dominance of positive feelings.

The basic principles of the Forgiveness Therapy indicated in this research are applied through the Inner Dialogue exercise. In the Inner Dialogue exercise, the activity of forgiveness is not only applied to the other person, but also to ourselves, as we take personal responsibility for our actions and our destiny. We require the activity of forgiving ourselves for our own personal development as much as the forgiving of the offending person.

13. Objective Compassion

It is said that love makes us blind to the failings of the cared one. But this can be expressed the other way round: love opens our eyes to the other's best qualities.

Rudolf Steiner (1861–1925)

In his *Curative Education Course,* Rudolf Steiner, the founder of Anthroposophy, introduced the concept of 'Objective Compassion,' a powerful attitude in education and therapy, and also very effective when applied to difficult social relationships.

Objective compassion allows us to heal ourselves and others from the impact of negative and extreme emotions, and unites two principles, which seem to contradict themselves: objectivity and compassion. Practising the HeartSpheres exercises can profoundly support the development of objective compassion and intuitive heart intelligence. (See Inner Dialogue, p.51.)

Contemporary life has brought immense challenges and risks for our physical, emotional, social and spiritual sanity. The need to practise these qualities has become ever more important for preventing and/or healing illness, and for empowering us within a rapidly changing and threatening environment.

Rudolf Steiner described the increasing need to create a new, self-regulated harmony between cognition, emotion and will. The importance of this is apparent: people and society increasingly show tendencies to veer either towards the pole of dry intellectualism, or unthinking action and aggression, both divorced from the mediating realm of feeling.

We can recognize these resulting pathologies easily:

Violence and hyperactivity are indications of a predominant will life too little governed by under-active thinking and perceiving, or by the appreciation and compassion of our weakened feelings.

Depression and anxiety are the result of a dominating cognitive life that overwhelms our feelings and our will and leads to passivity, indecision and emotional paralysis. We may develop obsessive-compulsive traits or fall prey to addiction.

The feelings and emotions may be too strong, clouding our common sense or forcing us into action, for example when we become fanatic and overbearing. We may become victims of severe mood swings.

Or we may suffer from shallowness of emotions, lack of enthusiasm and enjoyment, and so on.

These are only a few examples of symptoms deriving from an imbalance between the three forces of cognition, emotion and will.

The HeartSpheres exercises offer an effective way to develop a new, harmonious relationship between cognition, feeling and will, and lay the foundations for preventing or treating the pathologies mentioned above.

Rudolf Steiner's understanding of the role of the breathing process and the human heart in managing extreme emotions and developing heart intelligence is one of the three roots of the HeartSpheres approach.

Conclusion

Facing our own negative extreme feelings — such as fear, anger, hatred and despair — with calmness and detachment allows us to develop an observer consciousness towards ourselves. This in turn can help ease the impact these feelings have on us, and will allow us to gain insight into our own nature without being overwhelmed by such feelings.

In a next step we can learn to accept our own and other people's emotional responses by developing a strong sense of compassion, supported by the meditative approach that the HeartSpheres method provides. By absorbing negative emotions into our heart we learn to accept each other in our entirety and forgive each other for our errors. In so doing, we end the game of blaming each other for our misfortune and stop the indifference. We rather take active responsibility for our own lives and our impact on other people. Responsibility means that we can move away from blaming ourselves and others for our good or bad fortune, and rather consider our life as part of ourselves and not just a sum of random experiences. An inner attitude of questioning may grow within us, questions about ourselves and others. We may ask ourselves: "What does this life event want to teach me? What are the lessons to be learned? How can I turn a difficult situation into a strengthening and development-enhancing event? What are my deeper aspirations in life? And how can I achieve them?"

As we apply the HeartSpheres exercises, we will increasingly experience life as a field of learning, in which we can acquire new skills and virtues. We realise that our personal and professional development can benefit from mastering the challenges of difficult life events.

As we use our imagination to mentally rehearse our own transformation we learn to trust in this potential and are ready to support our own and other people's personal development. This creates the potential for personal change. We develop new interpersonal and professional skills and learn to put them into action. As we change ourselves, we will experience that our relationships and our life changes for the better too. We become more creative in our life and learn how to manifest our life aims and aspirations. The HeartSpheres exercises are powerful tools that allow us to live our lives to the full, with passion, enthusiasm and confidence, but always in consideration of our fellow human beings. As we continue to practise the exercises, we will learn to develop our ever growing capacity and potential for intuitive insight and understanding, care and compassion and inner strength and confidence.

These HeartSpheres qualities you can acquire are not sentimental, but real, strong and ... life-changing. You can gradually master your emotional response, which will lead to a strengthening of confidence and power, and ultimately to the mastery of your own will and the realization of your life aims. The HeartSpheres exercises can help you to take charge of your life and practise full presence of mind, by drawing on the strength, caring and growing intuitive intelligence of the heart.

14. The HeartSpheres Approach: Promoting Health and Enhancing Performance

Why do we need stress management?

We live in a culture of change, deadlines and increasing challenges. At the workplace, we must learn to work as a team despite competition and job insecurity. The financial markets have taken a turn for the worse, threatening economic downturn, even recession and inflation, with a potential knock-on effect on our individual financial security and our standard of living. At home we are threatened by the break-up of traditional family structures, long working hours, and the risks associated with young people growing up in an increasingly hostile environment. We are exposed to human conflicts never imagined before.

Although stress enhances performance initially, chronic and increasing levels of stress can make us more susceptible to physical and emotional illness (such as anxiety disorder and depression), burn-out and premature ageing. It impacts negatively on judgement, performance and decision-making.

As we need physical and emotional health and high performance to sustain our quality of life, we need to think about techniques that can help us develop the skills that allow us to sustain health, high performance and productivity.

The effective management of stress at home and at work is essential if you want to make the most of your potential. It will also help avoid the disruptive consequences of emotional stress, such as illness, unemployment, low commitment, failure to achieve goals, indecision and lack of enjoyment.

How does this approach promote emotional and physical health and good performance?

HeartSpheres actively promotes emotional and physical health and wellbeing, giving you tools and techniques to transform negative conditions, such as stress and anxiety, into positive actions to succeed in our increasingly stressful world.

We provide techniques based on a deep understanding of the physiology of the breathing process, the unity of the actions of heart and the brain, and their relationship to human consciousness and positive self-development. It is this proven connection between physiology and psychology that makes our exercises so effective.

These exercises not only *enhance skills and our performance* but also have a *profound health-promoting and illness-preventing effect.*

As we begin to manage our emotional responses and our breathing process, we learn to balance our autonomic nervous system, restore and enhance the regenerative power of our organism, and learn to prevent serious illness despite being exposed to extreme circumstances.

What are these techniques and are they easy to learn?

Autonomic nervous system balance, enhanced regeneration and health promotion are achieved by applying easily learned and powerful self-help techniques that employ a medically developed, Balanced Breathing technique. Once mastered, the Balanced Breathing technique can then be applied in conjunction with effective mental and emotional management techniques such as focused relaxation, visualization techniques, positive self-talk, and creating and sustaining positive feelings.

The HeartSpheres approach has developed very effective and

easy-to-learn techniques that can profoundly change our ability to cope with extreme or stressful circumstances and extreme emotions. The powerful techniques are easy to practise within a busy and challenging working and home environment.

What does HeartSpheres mean?

The name HeartSpheres reflects the harmonising of the three spheres of cognition, emotion and will. Balance between them ensures lasting capacity to proactively manage extreme emotions and stress both in the short and long term. This balancing is achieved through heart focus, regulated breathing and imagination techniques.

What is the scientific basis of these techniques?

We utilize emotional management tools, based on groundbreaking scientific research, to achieve the transformation from negative to positive emotional states. These techniques are effective and easy for all to master.

Dr. Peter Gruenewald, MD and his team developed the HeartSpheres approach and its techniques based on scientific research in the field of chronobiology (chronobiological medicine) and positive (motivational) psychology.

What is chronobiological medicine?

Chronobiology is the science of biological rhythms and their influence on illness and health.

Severe illnesses like heart disease, hypertension, diabetes and cancer are accompanied by pathological changes in biological rhythms in their early preventable state. These changes in biological rhythm include disturbances to sleeping and waking patterns as well as changes in breathing and circulation (heart rhythms). Such rhythmic disruption is the concern of chronobiology, which is defined as the effect of time in living systems.

The cutting edge advances in chronobiological research, notably researches on *heart-rate variability*, have led to the development of diagnostic and therapeutic approaches, which are of value not only in effective health promotion, but also in the treatment and prevention of disease. Heart-rate variability measures the changing intervals between two heartbeats. Today, heart-rate variability is a scientifically recognized tool to measure autonomic nervous-system function.

The autonomic nervous system regulates the function and rhythm of all organs, particularly the relationship between breathing and circulation or heart function. It comprises two opposite players: the sympathetic and the parasympathetic systems. The sympathetic autonomic nervous system is responsible for the well-known 'fight or flight' response, when we have to be alert — as in an emergency situation. The parasympathetic autonomic nervous system, as its corresponding counterpart, is responsible for relaxation, regeneration, nutrition and sleep.

The autonomic nervous system also has a close connection with our endocrine and immune systems, for example via the function of the suprarenal glands in releasing adrenalin, cortisol or DHEA.

If our autonomic nervous system is in a functional balance then we are capable of recovering from any stress or strain without suffering any ill effects. If the system is out of balance, we will start to become susceptible to ill health such as hypertension, heart disease, diabetes, infectious diseases, cancer and premature ageing.

One factor that strongly influences the balance of our autonomic nervous system is our emotions. We know now that a vast number of medical conditions are caused by the influence of strong negative emotions on our biorhythms and our autonomic nervous system. We also know that positive emotions, on the other hand, have a harmonizing and thereby health-promoting effect on our body.

Measuring heart-rate variability gives an accurate picture of the ability of the organism to recover from stress and strain, and allows us to measure the impact of lifestyle and emotions on our general health.

Maintaining a high level and good coherence of heart-rate variability means that the heart has the capacity to vary its heartbeat given different conditions of stress and strain, and recover from them. With a high level and coherence of heart-rate variability, the autonomic nervous system is in a balanced state, thus enhancing cognitive function which includes *concentration, focus, memory, flexibility of response, intuitive insight, judgement and decision-making.*

As we grow older, heart-rate variability reduces naturally. Heart-rate variability is an indicator of the relative youthfulness of our organism, its power of regeneration, its adaptability and flexibility. Heart-rate variability reduces with negative chronic stress. Thus, a low level of heart-rate variability indicates that an individual is at risk of developing a serious illness or is ageing prematurely. Scientific research has shown that heart-rate variability is an accurate predictor of the likelihood of sudden cardiac and even non-cardiac death and of the risk of accidents.

HeartSpheres exercises increase heart-rate variability and coherence immediately and in the long term. This health improvement can be monitored. We measure heart-rate variability in our clients by means of heart-balance technology called HeartMan®. The HeartMan is a 24-hour ECG holster that measures and registers fine changes within the heart and breathing rhythm. This produces a so-called auto-chronic image (ACI) that can be interpreted in cooperation with the health professional to give an accurate picture of the ability of the organism to recover from stress and strain. The result also indicates sleep quality and vitality and indicates a potential risk of ill health, thus contributing to illness prevention.

This technology is used to monitor the health progress of an individual while pursuing HeartSpheres exercises or a wellness programme.

The HeartMan technology was developed by Professor Dr. Max Moser, human physiologist at the University of Graz, Austria and is widely used in research, executive coaching, rehabilitation and sports medicine.

What is the physiological effect of the HeartSpheres techniques?

Scientific research has shown that combining these positive emotional states with controlled breathing has the following short- and long-term physiological effects:

Balancing the autonomic nervous system:

~ Sympathetic ('fight and flight' response – states of heightened alertness and mobilized energy) and parasympathetic (relaxation and regeneration) activity are balanced during a state of focused relaxation. This newly achieved balance in the function of the autonomic nervous system results in improvement and possibly prevention of stress-related diseases, such as high blood pressure, coronary heart disease, asthma, irritable bowel syndrome and insomnia.

Harmonizing the endocrine system:

~ Focused relaxation, combined with positive emotional states and controlled breathing has been shown to affect the endocrine system. The blood levels of stress hormones dopamine, adrenaline and cortisol are reduced and the level of the youth hormone Dehydroepiandrosterone (DHEA) is increased. (DHEA is a natural hormone produced from cholesterol by the adrenal glands, the gonads, adipose tissue, brain and the skin.)

The reduction of stress hormones and the increase of DHEA have the following effects:

~ Reduced insulin resistance (reduction of the risk of developing type 2 diabetes)

~ Improved moods and relief from depression

~ Improved fat metabolism (reduced cholesterol and triglycerides, prevention of associated illnesses, such as coronary heart disease)

~ Increased immune system function (reduced number and duration of infections, improved recovery)

~ Slows down the ageing process

~ Increased lean muscle mass

~ A direct causal relationship of increased levels of DHEA and reduced levels of cortisol on certain conditions has been postulated and is currently the subject of research. These conditions include cardiovascular disease, diabetes, hypercholesterolemia, obesity, multiple sclerosis, Parkinson's disease, Alzheimer's disease, disorders of the immune system, depression, osteoporosis and some sexual dysfunctions.

~ Modulating the immune system — there are strong indications that practising the HeartSpheres exercises has a directly beneficial influence on the immune system, improving allergies and increasing resistance to infections.

What is applied positive psychology?

Applied positive psychology *"focuses on the strengths and virtues that enable individuals and communities to thrive."* Positive psychologists seek *"to find and nurture genius and talent,"* and *"to make normal life more fulfilling,"* not to cure mental illness.

Negative extreme emotions impact negatively on professional and private human relationships. Although we can manage our exposure to stress, often to a very limited degree, the main question remains: *How do we change the way we process stressful events and activities so that we can utilize the energy behind extreme emotions* (anxiety, fear, frustration etc.) *without being affected negatively in health and performance?*

The HeartSpheres techniques were developed to *promote physical and emotional health* and to *enhance performance in a stressful environment*. Although it is fully acknowledged that stress and extreme emotions can have a positive impact on enhancing performance, this is only a short-term advantage. Prolonged and high levels of stress eventually take their toll on health and performance.

Practising the exercises regularly enables one to *achieve and sustain a positive emotional state* (such as calmness, appreciation and/or confidence) not only during the exercises, but also *during challenging life situations*.

What is the psychological effect of the HeartSpheres techniques?

The psychological effects are:
~ Reduced intensity of disturbing emotions, such as anxiety, fear, irritability, anger, frustration and depression.

~ Enhanced interpersonal skills, such as better listening, patience, initiative and leadership.

~ Improved creative problem solving through enhanced emotional intelligence.

~ Better decision-making and performance.

~ Overall, our thinking, feeling and will capacities work in better harmony with each other and our social environment.

After reading this book, where can I go for further HeartSpheres training?

Reading and working with this book will empower you to practise these exercises on your own. You may nevertheless want to deepen the experience of these exercises by undergoing individual or group coaching with the help of a qualified HeartSpheres trainer.

A licensed HeartSpheres trainer provides HeartSpheres training and coaching. They are trained and supervised by a medical doctor and GP with a special interest in chronobiology and applied positive psychology.

What should I expect from individual coaching sessions?

Individual coaching includes a careful review of your personal and medical history, as well as an assessment of current and future health risks. It may include further lifestyle advice (such as dietary measures) and a physical exercise programme and may, if applicable, be complemented by other therapeutic interventions or life-skill coaching.

How do we evaluate any progress while practising the exercises?

HeartSpheres trainers utilize emotional management tools based on groundbreaking scientific research, which documents the transformation from negative to positive emotional states and the balancing of the autonomic nervous system.

As described above, measuring heart-rate variability (HRV) and its coherence facilitates evaluation of the effect of the autonomic nervous system activity on heart and circulation. A high heart-rate variability is found in youthful states of health: it is high in childhood and decreases with age and poor health. Low heart-rate variability has been shown to be an accurate predictor of a person's state of health. Coherence is another reliable indicator for autonomic nervous system balance. High coherence and high heart-rate variability indicate effective stress-relief and the presence of an equally focused and relaxed state of mind.

The long-term efficacy of the HeartSpheres exercises is measured as follows:

The HeartMan®

~ A 24 hour ECG is performed by the HeartMan®, which uses heart-rate variability as a diagnostic tool for the (short- and long-term) impact of stress on the organism. The HeartMan has been developed and researched by Professor Max Moser, a medical physiologist at the University of Graz, Austria.

~ Medical measurements conducted on cosmonauts in space, which the Russian space medicine group invited for 9 missions (Austro-Mir project), were the starting point of the HeartMan project.

~ The HeartMan creates an Autochrone Image (ACI) resulting from monitoring HRV and other rhythms throughout the day and night. This facilitates objective evaluation of the degree of stress during daily activity, the quality of sleep via ECG measurements and a person's fitness. This test likewise objectively evaluates the efficacy of stress management techniques, therapies, preventive medical treatments and lifestyle changes. The test results can also motivate people to change their lifestyle.

The Depression Anxiety and Stress Scale (DASS)

~ The outcome of the HeartSpheres coaching is audited using a questionnaire called the Depression Anxiety Stress Scale (DASS) developed in Australia. The DASS has been standardized for worldwide use and is a recognized psychological assessment tool. Prior to the HeartSpheres training, the client fills in an assessment questionnaire consisting of 48 simple questions. After practising the Heartspheres exercises for four weeks, the questionnaire is again completed in order to monitor progress and outcome.

Personal evaluation
~ A means of evaluating your own progress is to keep an exercise diary. Define your developmental aims (what you would like to achieve) and determine a suitable time to review the results of your exercises. Take note of the difficulties you encountered when practising the exercises, and try to develop strategies for improving your skills and overcoming any difficulties or obstacles.

Is it possible to arrange group workshops for businesses?

HeartSpheres Ltd provides workshops for businesses, charities, health professionals and any organization which considers their members' development, health and performance as important. These workshops are tailored to the specific needs and questions of the organizations. All workshops are experiential and interactive.

You can also attend one of our group workshops, which are held regularly in the UK and worldwide. For more information on workshops for organizations and the public, please visit the HeartSpheres Ltd website: *www. heartspheres.com*

Individual coaching is also provided at the Hale Clinic, London, and at the Helios Medical Centre, Bristol. For more information visit our website: *www.regenerativehealthclinic.net*

Bibliography and Further Reading

Bott, Victor (2004) *Introduction to Anthroposophical Medicine — Extending the Art of Healing,* Anthroposophic Press, USA.

Childre, Doc, & Rozman, Deborah (2006) *Transforming Anxiety: The HeartMath Solution for Overcoming Fear and Worry and Creating Serenity,* New Harbinger Publications, USA.

Childre, Doc & Martin, Howard (2000) *The HeartMath Solution: The Institute of HeartMath's Revolutionary Program for Engaging the Power of the Heart's Intelligence,* HarperSanFrancisco, USA.

Childre, Doc & Cryer, B (1999) *From Chaos to Coherence: Advancing Emotional and Organizational Intelligence Through Inner Quality Management,* Butterworth-Heinemann, USA

Csikszentmihalyi, Mihaly (2002) *Flow: The Classic Work on How to Achieve Happiness,* Rider & Co., UK.

Gottman, John (1995) *Why Marriages Succeed or Fail: And How You Can Make Yours Last,* Simon & Schuster.

Gruenewald, Dr Peter (2001) *Gold and the Philosopher's Stone: Treating Chronic Physical and Mental Illness With Mineral Remedies,* Temple Lodge, UK.

Lehrs, Ernst (1985) *Man and Matter,* Rudolf Steiner Press, UK.

Linden, Wolfgang (2005) *Stress Management — From Basic Science to Better Practice,* Sage Publications, USA.

Lipson, Michael (2002) *Stairway of Surprise, Six Steps to a Creative Life,* Anthroposophic Press, USA.

Pearce, Stewart (2006) *The Alchemy of Voice,* Hodder Mobius, UK.

Rosenberg, Marshall B. (2003) *Nonviolent Communication: A Language of Life — Create Your Life, Your Relationships, and Your World in Harmony with Your Values,* 2nd edition, Puddledancer Press, USA.

Servan-Schreiber, David, (2003) *Healing without Freud and Prozac,* Rodale, USA.

Steiner, Rudolf (1998) *Education for Special Needs, The Curative Education Course, Twelve Lectures,* Dornach, June 25–July 7, 1924, Rudolf Steiner Press, UK.

—, (1995) *Intuitive Thinking as a Spiritual Path: A Philosophy of Freedom,* Steiner Books, USA.

—, (1994) *How to Know Higher Worlds: A Modern Path of Initiation,* Anthroposophic Press, USA.